About the Autł .ــ.

Dr Marilyn Glenville PhD is the UK's leading nutritionist specialising in women's health. She obtained her doctorate from Cambridge University and is a fellow of the Royal Society of Medicine.

Dr Glenville is the former president of the Food and Health Forum at the Royal Society of Medicine and is patron of the Daisy Network, a premature menopause charity.

For more than 40 years, Dr Glenville has studied and practised nutrition, both in the UK and in the USA. She gives lectures and seminars throughout the world and appears regularly on radio and TV.

Dr Glenville has written 14 internationally best-selling books which have sold over one million copies worldwide and have been translated into 20 languages.

The Books Include;

Natural Alternatives to Sugar, Fat Around the Middle - and How to Get Rid of it, Natural Solutions to the Menopause, Osteoporosis - How to Prevent, Treat and Reverse it, Healthy Eating for the Menopause, Natural Solutions to PCOS, Natural Solutions to IBS, Getting Pregnant Faster, Overcoming PMS the Natural Way, The Natural Health Bible for Women, The Nutritional Health Handbook for Women.

Dr Glenville has won the Best Nutrition Health Writer of the Year ٫ard and has also been awarded a place in the current edition of ٛo's Who of famous people.

Dr Glenville runs clinics in Harley Street in London, Tunbridge ׀ls in Kent and Dublin, Galway, Cork and Kilkenny in Ireland (see ׀ ٛources page at back of book). Her website is www.marilynglenville.

׀ .

Acknowledgements

As mentioned in the introduction, this book has been a rather personal journey because Alzheimer's has directly affected my family. It has been a revelation to look at the amount of research on diet and lifestyle, in relation to dementia and Alzheimer's, and to think that many people may not get to hear about this vital information that could help them.

I would like to thank Karen Evennett for helping to make sure that this book is easy to read and to Judy Barratt for structuring the book so that it flows well. And to Donna Gambazza for managing the logistics in the background.

I would also like to thank all the nutritionists who work with me in the UK: Anna Firth, Helen Ford, Sally Milne, Sharon Pitt and Lisa Smith and those in Ireland, headed by Heather Leeson and Ciara Wright, and also Sorcha Molloy in Galway. And to Jessie Anderson my clinic manager and her team, Annabel Bolton and Lucy Fordyce.

Last but not least, my love goes to my family: Kriss, my husband, and my three children Matt (and his wife Hannah and their children Katie and Jack), Len (and Mel) and Chantell.

Dedication

To my father (Alec) and mother-in-law (Eva)
who both died from dementia.

And to you dear reader who wants to stay mentally
and physically bright and healthy as you grow
into your golden years

Natural Solutions for Dementia and Alzheimer's

Your 7-Step Brain Protection Plan

Dr Marilyn Glenville PhD

Natural Solutions for Dementia and Alzheimer's -
Your 7-Step Brain Protection Plan

Dr Marilyn Glenville PhD

First published in the United Kingdom and Ireland in 2017 by Lifestyles Press
14 St John's Road, Tunbridge Wells, Kent TN4 9NP

Conceived, created and designed by Lifestyles Press 2017
Production Manager: Donna Gambazza, Lifestyles Press
Managing Designer: Sian Collins, www.siancollins-designer.com
British Library Cataloguing-in-Publication Data:
A CIP record for this book is available from the British Library

ISBN: 978-0-9935431-6-6

Typeset in ITC Garamond BT
Printed in UK

Disclaimer: The contents of this book are for information only and are intended
to assist readers in identifying symptoms and conditions they may be experiencing.
This book is not intended to be a substitute for taking proper medical advice and
should not be relied upon in this way. Always consult a qualified doctor or health
practitioner. The author and publisher cannot accept responsibility for illness
arising out of the failure to seek medical advice from a doctor.

Contents

Introduction

Three things happen as you get older. The first is your memory goes – and I can't remember the other two. That famous Norman Wisdom joke tickles us all – but it's not such a laughing matter when memory loss starts to become a reality. Could it, we worry, be the first sign of Alzheimer's or dementia? I have to admit that this has not been an easy book for me to write. In doing so, I have realised that Alzheimer's or dementia has affected most of us (myself included) in some way; and it is a painful process. Many of you reading this book will be concerned about relatives who may already be displaying symptoms; or, perhaps, they have already been diagnosed. Others of you may know that you have a strong family history of dementia and Alzheimer's and that you need to start thinking about what changes you can make in your life to reduce your chances of developing the condition yourself.

There is a light at the end of the tunnel. Even though the medical world has not been very successful at treating dementia and Alzheimer's, nutritional and lifestyle interventions have – but you have probably not heard about them! Unfortunately, unlike developing and selling a drug – a magic cure-all – patented by a pharmaceutical company, there is no big money in getting someone to change their diet.

The result is that the information that could help so many people gets buried. And, because that information doesn't make the headlines, the people who really need it – the sufferers and their carers, and all those who are potential sufferers – don't get to know about what we can do to help ourselves or those close to us.

I have written this book to share with you all the latest scientific research showing what we can do to help ourselves in a practical way to either prevent or reverse the decline in cognitive function that is caused by dementia and Alzheimer's.

For any health problem, effective treatment begins with understanding the cause. Whether you suffer from IBS, irregular periods, PCOS, or dementia or Alzheimer's, preventing or treating the underlying triggers is more powerful than merely papering over the symptoms.

In order to help unravel what might trigger cognitive malfunction, I start the book by explaining the difference between dementia and Alzheimer's, as often the two terms are used interchangeably but they are not the same. I have looked at how many people are affected by Alzheimer's and the theories behind its causes. We'll ask; is Alzheimer's a genetic issue? Does family history predispose us to it? And, if so, can we do anything about it? We'll look at what research reveals about how nutritional choices can affect dementia and Alzheimer's. Do particular vitamins and minerals help with slowing or reversing the progression of memory decline? We'll look at whether it really makes a difference if we use games to stimulate brain activity or whether this is just the sales patter of app developers. And what about exercise? We know it is important for physical health, but what does the research show when it comes to the effect of exercise on our mental wellbeing?

Even though writing this book has touched a personal nerve (my father and mother-in-law developed Alzheimer's and I saw first hand the effects not only on them, but on all those who had to care for them), my research has shown me just how much we do know already and how very beneficial simple, practical lifestyle changes can be, not only to help prevent the disease but also to slow the decline for those who already have it.

I hope you find the information in the book as interesting as I did while I was gathering it; and I hope that it can make a difference both to you and to your family.

PART ONE

UNDERSTANDING DEMENTIA

Chapter 1

Understanding your memory

You may have heard that your mind can be thought of as a filing cabinet full of individual folders, each one holding a memory that's stored away for safekeeping until you need it. But, of course, the way your memory works is really far more complex than that.

For a start, your memory is not just in one particular place in your brain – instead it is a brain-wide process, with different areas of your brain working together to form what we call memory. For example, riding a bike involves the memory of how to operate the bicycle, which is stored in one area of the brain, together with the memory of the route you need to follow, which is stored in another. From another area, your memory needs to locate the rules of the road, while – from yet another area – you will remember that anxious feeling when a vehicle veers dangerously close to you.

Each element of a memory – including sights, sounds, words, smells, physical feelings and emotions – is stored in the same part of the brain that originally created that fragment (the visual cortex, motor cortex, the area that controls language and so on). When you recall a memory, you reactivate the neural patterns that were generated during the original encoding. Adding to the complexity, your brain encodes and stores short– and long–term memories in different ways and in separate parts of your brain.

So, rather than thinking of memories as individual files in a cabinet, it may be better to think of them as separate threads in a complex, interconnected web. Every thread of memory intersects and crosses other memories to create a rounded 'whole' web of memory. Or you might prefer to think of your memory as a jigsaw puzzle, with lots of tiny pieces that all need to link up before an individual memory can be formed. When we think about memory in these ways, it is easy to see how, even when part of the brain is damaged, some memories – or fragments of memories – remain.

This book investigates what goes wrong with the brain when a person develops dementia and Alzheimer's and what we can do to protect our memory function when that happens. The good news is that not every memory problem is something to worry about.

Thanks for the memories

The different things you remember – events, facts or skills – are all stored and recalled by different types of memory working together.

- **Declarative memory** is what you use when you remember a place, name fact or event.
- **Procedural memory** involves those learned habits you've known and used for years, such as tying your shoelaces or riding a bike.
- **Episodic memory** is specific to you and recalls specific things you have done – for example, who you met, what you said and what you did on a certain day.
- **Semantic memory** is your general knowledge about the world around you. For example, you know that acorns grow on oak trees.

What's normal, what's not?

Chances are that you have had the common experience of wandering purposefully into a room, only to come to a grinding halt because you suddenly can't remember why you went there. You may have also forgotten the name of the celebrity at the centre of a story you're trying to tell. Or you may mislay your keys, forget occasional appointments or sometimes return from the shops without one or two of the things you'd gone for. You may read a passage from a book, and then realise you haven't taken in a word…

When these things happen in your twenties, you can joke about them but, as you age, memory lapses are not such a laughing matter. If they seem to be happening more frequently than they have before, you may worry that they could be the early signs of dementia or Alzheimer's – serious conditions involving ever-deteriorating memory. You may worry with good reason, too; age is the number one risk factor for dementia and Alzheimer's. It is not that growing older *causes* dementia and Alzheimer's but that, as you age, these conditions become more likely. According to figures supplied by Age UK in 2014, of the estimated 850,000 people who were living with dementia in the UK, 773,502 were aged 65 and over.

Dementia and Alzheimer's disease provide the focus of this book and it's important to reassure you, right at the outset, that being forgetful is often *not* a sign of either. Furthermore, although we are likely to become more forgetful as we get older, in most cases simple forgetfulness will not be the start of the kind of mental decline that is characteristic of dementia.

Yes, your memory is likely to malfunction with age; and, yes, minor lapses are likely to become more noticeable. However, these are usually owing to normal changes in the structure and function of the ageing brain, which (like all the other parts of your body) is subject to the normal physical decline – such as shrinking, slowing and stiffening – associated with advancing years.

But how do we quantify 'normal' decline in memory function against what might be a sign of something more sinister? Although often alarming, the following are all considered normal. They may become more pronounced as you age, but they are not usually thought to be indicative of dementia, unless they are extreme and persistent.

Transience

This is the tendency to forget facts soon after learning them, or information or events over time. Although worrying when it happens – especially if you haven't been used to it happening before – it is not usually the sign of memory weakness that you may imagine. In fact, if you think of your mind as a house filled with those memory cobwebs, every now and then it needs a spring clean to keep it fresh and allow space for new webs to form. It's also unlikely that the memories you most need – and use most frequently – are the ones you'll lose. Non-essential information, therefore, gets swept away.

Absentmindedness

This is what happens when you don't focus on the thing you are doing, because your mind is occupied with something that you have given greater priority. So, you may forget where you put your pen or your spectacles because when you put them down you were focusing on something else. Things you do every day, as part of a routine, can also suffer when you are absentminded. For example, you may take a medicine at the same point in your morning routine every day so that taking it becomes second nature. As a result, you could very well be thinking about something else when you pop that pill. Later, when you focus on the fact that you were supposed to take your medicine, you might not actually remember doing so. This is one of the reasons why so many long-term-usage drugs come in blister packets labelled with the days of the week.

There are many reasons why we may become absentminded in the first place, of course – being overworked or generally too busy, trying to juggle the demands of a family and/or a job, or feeling stressed about something in particular that's going on in your life are all causes of absentmindedness. If any of those scenarios could apply to you, try to take stock and think of ways that you could reduce activity and/or stress in your life to bring back some focus (see pp.132–140).

Tip-of-the-tongue syndrome

Whether you're trying to keep up with *University Challenge* or *Pointless*, you may be 100 per cent sure of the answer to that million-dollar question, but you just can't retrieve the right words. While that might be hugely frustrating, it's nothing to worry about. Memory specialists call having something on the tip-of-the-tongue 'blocking' and it occurs when a competing and very similar memory pops up so intrusively that you are prevented from locating the actual memory you're after. Blocking is more likely to occur when you're tired and especially when you're trying to remember proper nouns. So common that most languages recognise it, the phenomenon is caused by a breakdown in the normal process by which the brain translates thoughts from abstract concepts into words to which it attaches the appropriate sounds. It sounds complicated, but actually that's a process that normally runs smoothly and easily. We don't yet fully understand why the process of retrieving the right piece of information becomes interrupted, but the word you're missing is likely to come back to you if someone gives you a clue, or if you find a clue yourself. Going through the alphabet could provide just the trigger you need to snap the word to mind.

Misattribution

Another kind of memory lapse that becomes more common with age, misattribution refers to remembering something accurately but only in part. For example, you may have what you think to be a crystal-clear memory of a particular event but, in fact, misattribute the time, location or person involved. Or you may come up with what you think to be an original thought of your own – when in fact it has come from something you've read or been told in the past. Old memories are especially likely to be subject to misattribution, but new memories formed during old age are also susceptible because, as we age, we find it increasingly difficult to concentrate on what we're experiencing or being told and to process information rapidly. However, misattribution is not a sign of dementia.

Suggestibility

Rather than forgetting or misremembering something, suggestibility is all to do with the power of suggestion, which fools your brain into thinking you remember something that was in fact information you learned after the event. For example, if you witnessed a car accident and later someone told you that one of the people involved was wearing a red coat, you could start to remember seeing the red coat – even though, in fact, you did not notice it at the time. In truth, the other witness may have been mistaken and there may not have been a red coat at all. Scientists still have a long way to go before fully understanding how the suggestibility is processed in the brain – but the result is to create a 'false' memory of something that doesn't exist or didn't happen at all.

Normal age-related memory loss doesn't prevent you from living a full and productive life. If you forget someone's name, you will probably recall it later in the day; and if you misplace your spectacles occasionally, or need to make lists more often than you've had to in the past, it's not the end of the world. These things don't disrupt your ability to work or maintain a normal, independent life.

When to worry

So, what are the signs that there is something to worry about? The following are all indications that your forgetfulness may have strayed beyond what wc considcr a normal part of the ageing process. This is especially true if any of these signs have started to happen a lot.

- Repeatedly asking the same questions.

- Forgetting common words when speaking.

- Mixing words up – saying 'bed' instead of 'table', for example.

- Taking longer to complete familiar tasks, such as following a recipe.

- Putting items in inappropriate places, such as putting a wallet in the fridge.

- Getting lost while walking or driving around a familiar neighbourhood.

- Undergoing sudden changes in mood or behaviour for no apparent reason.

- Becoming less able to follow directions.

Increasing forgetfulness, alongside changes in your ability to concentrate and pay attention, and a slowing down of the speed with which you can process information may be signs of mild cognitive impairment – but this shouldn't normally interfere with your life or prevent you from carrying out usual activities. Mild cognitive impairment can sometimes progress to Alzheimer's or dementia, but not always. You can develop mild cognitive impairment without your memory loss progressing and without developing the whole spectrum of symptoms associated with dementia. It is an area of research that doctors still have much to learn about.

No going back?

Mild cognitive impairment does not always become more severe. In some cases, its worsening can stop and cognitive function may even begin to improve. There are many reversible causes of memory loss and impaired cognitive function – including:

- **Medications**, either individually or in combination.

- **Minor head trauma or injury** – even if it doesn't result in a loss of consciousness – from a fall or accident.

- **Depression or other mental health disorders**, including stress and anxiety.

- **Chronic alcoholism** either as a result of the addiction and its physical effects itself, or as a result of the interaction of the alcohol with medications you may be taking.

- **Vitamin B12 deficiency**, which means that the body lacks a nutrient that is essential to the health of nerve cells and red blood cells. B12 deficiency is particularly common among older adults.

- **Hypothyroidism (underactive thyroid)**, which slows the processing (metabolism) of nutrients to create energy for cells.

- **Tumour** in the brain.

Although some of the entries on this list may seem scary, with diagnosis most of these conditions are perfectly treatable and effective treatment will restore your normal memory or cognitive function. And, if memory function is poor as a result of a non-definable medical condition, perhaps because you are simply too busy to concentrate properly or generally under the weather, there is plenty you can do through your lifestyle choices to keep your mental acuity in peak condition for as long as the natural ageing process allows.

Chapter 2

Diagnosing dementia

The terms dementia and Alzheimer's are often used interchangeably but dementia is actually an umbrella term for up to 100 different types of disease, of which Alzheimer's disease is just one. What's more, a person can suffer with more than one of form at any one time. I'm going to start this chapter by outlining some of the most common forms of dementia we know about and, to do that, first we need to understand a bit about the brain and how it works.

Brain matters

Each part of your brain has a different function. The type of dementia a person suffers from depends upon which brain function has become impaired – that is, which part of the brain has become diseased. The main brain parts and functions are:

- **The brain stem**, at the base of the brain, which controls your automatic body functions such as heartbeat and breathing.

- **The cerebellum**, which is responsible for your balance and posture.

- **The limbic system**, which lies deep inside the brain, includes the hippocampus (the key to your memory) and the amygdala (which plays a vital role in your emotional health).

- **The cerebrum**, which comprises the cerebral hemispheres that make up three-quarters of the whole brain. The cerebrum is responsible for consciousness, memory, reasoning, language and social skills. The left cerebral hemisphere is responsible for language; while the right governs our understanding of where we are in relation to the things around us.

- **The cortex**, which is a thin layer of grey matter covering the cerebrum and containing billions of brain cells. Beneath the grey matter of the cortex is white matter, which is made up of bundles of nerve fibres. These fibres transport nerve signals between parts of the cortex and from the cortex to other parts of the brain.

- **The lobes**, which are located in the cerebrum. Examples of the functions of your lobes, and how impairment might manifest itself in dementia are given below.

The lobes and their functions

There are four lobes (occipital, temporal, parietal and frontal) in each cerebral hemisphere. Each one has its own vital role to play, as well as working with the other lobes.

- **The occipital lobes** at the back of the brain deal with visual information (damage in this area can, therefore, cause blindness).

- **The parietal lobes**, in the upper-rear part of the cerebrum, handle information from your other senses and enable you to know how to pick up a fork to eat with, or to put one leg in front of the other to walk. You use your left parietal lobe to read, write and process numbers, while your right parietal lobe helps you to recognise objects as being three-dimensional. Alzheimer's often involves damage to the left parietal lobe, which may lead to problems with, say, getting dressed; damage to the right parietal lobe can prevent you from recognising where you are, causing you to get lost.

- **The temporal lobes**, on either side of your brain (near your temples), are themselves divided up into sections that govern different brain functions. The hippocampus lies inside the temporal lobes either side of your brain. This briefly stores the patterns of neurons that make up a memory before passing them along to the parts of the brain that will preserve them for the long term. Therefore, the hippocampus is crucial for forming new memories. The outer part of each temporal lobe is where you store your general knowledge – known as semantic memory. Again, the different sides deal with different things. The left stores facts, word meanings and names of objects, while the right stores the visual memories that help you to recognise familiar faces and objects.

- **The frontal lobes** form the large and complex management centre of your brain, helping you to solve problems and make decisions. You use this management centre to follow the steps of a familiar task, such as making a piece of toast and buttering it. It also helps you to keep focused on a single task and to learn new and complex skills until they become automatic – like learning to drive. The effects of damage to the frontal lobes depends upon on which area is affected. For example, if the part of your frontal lobe to do with motivation is damaged you could become apathetic and reluctant to engage with life. Alternatively, if there is damage to the part of your frontal lobe that governs social behaviour, you could become disinhibited, saying or doing inappropriate things. Finally, damage to the motor cortex, at the back of the frontal lobes, causes problems with moving and controlling certain muscles – so you may, for example, have trouble clapping your hands or (if the damage is to the control mechanisms for your jaw muscles) even smiling or speaking.

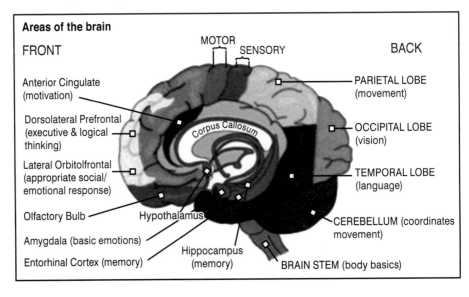

Areas of the brain

FRONT — MOTOR SENSORY — BACK

Anterior Cingulate (motivation)

Dorsolateral Prefrontal (executive & logical thinking)

Lateral Orbitolfrontal (appropriate social/ emotional response)

Corpus Callosum

Olfactory Bulb — Hypothalamus

Amygdala (basic emotions)

Entorhinal Cortex (memory)

Hippocampus (memory)

PARIETAL LOBE (movement)

OCCIPITAL LOBE (vision)

TEMPORAL LOBE (language)

CEREBELLUM (coordinates movement)

BRAIN STEM (body basics)

Alzheimer's disease

Accounting for 50 to 75 per cent of cases, Alzheimer's disease is the most common form of dementia. Caused by plaques and tangles developing in the brain, Alzheimer's kills more people in the USA each year than breast and prostate cancer combined. I'll discuss Alzheimer's in more detail in the next chapter.

Frontotemporal dementia

The second most common cause of dementia in the under-65s, but less common in older people, frontotemporal dementia is caused when abnormal proteins prevent the brain cells from communicating with each other as they should. One-third of cases are thought to be genetic. Symptoms may include: personality changes, repetitive behaviour, changes in appetite (which can lead to uncharacteristic binge-eating), and difficulties with decision making, problem solving and concentration. Some sufferers may experience problems with speech – for example, losing an understanding of familiar words – as well as difficulties recognising objects and people. Frontotemporal dementia can cause uninhibited and inappropriate behaviour in public. This form of dementia may be confused with depression, psychosis or obsessive compulsive disorder.

Dementia with Lewy bodies

The third most common cause of dementia, usually occurring in people over the age of 65 years (people over the age of 80 have a one-in-six chance of developing Lewy bodies), Lewy bodies dementia accounts for about 15 per cent of all dementia cases. Lewy bodies are clumps of proteins that develop in the nerve cells. These damage nerve-cell function and inhibit the way the cells communicate with one another.

Like all forms of dementia, this is a progressive condition, with symptoms (which can be similar to those of both Alzheimer's and Parkinson's) gradually worsening over time. Common symptoms include fluctuating alertness and concentration levels, confusion, mood changes, difficulty with everyday tasks, problems with spatial awareness, a decline in problem-solving skills, slowed movement and stiffness, tremors, restlessness, unsteadiness and increased falls. Furthermore, the nerve-cell damage that occurs as a result of Lewy bodies can cause hallucinations – you could hear things or see things that are not there. Interestingly, memory is often less affected than with other types of dementia, but you might experience sudden bouts of confusion. People with Lewy bodies also tend to fall asleep easily during the day, but then have disturbed sleep at night, including experiencing intense dreams and nightmares.

There are certain risk factors that can make us more likely to develop dementia with Lewy bodies. These include:

- Gender: twice as many women as men over the age of 65 are diagnosed with dementia with Lewy bodies.

- Genetics: in rare cases, and usually in people under the age of 65, dementia with Lewy bodies can be passed from one generation to another.

- Poor physical health or inadequately controlled physical disorders, such as diabetes or heart disease.

- Poor lifestyle choices, such as smoking, lack of exercise and excessive use of alcohol.

Vascular dementia

Causing between 20 and 30 per cent of dementia cases, but rarely seen in the under-65s, vascular dementia is another umbrella term. The word vascular means 'relating to blood vessels', so someone with vascular dementia will be suffering with a problem to do with blood supply (and, therefore, oxygen) to the brain. There are several causes for impeded blood flow, including small clots (sometimes known as transient ischemic attacks or TIAs) that damage the blood vessels, blocked arteries (atherosclerosis) and burst blood vessels (haemorrhages). You're at greater risk of vascular dementia if you have a family history of stroke, heart disease or diabetes – in fact, if you also go on to develop any of these conditions, your risk of developing vascular dementia doubles.

Smoking, drinking excessively and poor physical fitness can also contribute to increased risk.

When TIAs are the underlying cause of vascular dementia, the small amount of recovery following a TIA can lead to the dementia appearing to get better for a while. However, because TIAs fundamentally damage the blood vessels, it is usually only a matter of time before dementia surfaces again and begins to cause ongoing problems with memory, decision making, daily living and so on.

Causes of dementia in the over-65s

This diagram illustrates the causes of dementia in the over-65s, from the most common (Alzheimer's) to the least common. It's important to remember that some of these causes may be more likely to occur in those who are younger.

Types of Dementia cases diagnosed in over 65s in the UK

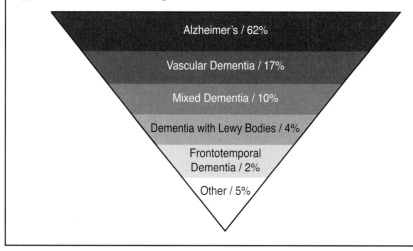

Alzheimer's / 62%

Vascular Dementia / 17%

Mixed Dementia / 10%

Dementia with Lewy Bodies / 4%

Frontotemporal Dementia / 2%

Other / 5%

Symptoms of dementia

We've touched briefly on the symptoms that each of the main forms of dementia may present and it's clear from these specific causes that loss of memory (usually short-term memory, so inability to retain new information) is just one symptom among many.

Looking at dementia in a more general sense, common symptoms include:

- **Disorientation.** This can relate to whereabouts (for example, relatives of people with dementia notice that their loved ones get lost in once familiar places) or to time of life (for example, some people with dementia may get up in the middle of the night and start dressing for work – even though they retired years before). Disorientation is to do with failing cognitive ability – the brain skills we normally use to solve problems are not as sharp as they once were. When cognitive ability starts to fail, reasoning, focus and concentration start to fail and we may become restless, preferring to keep doing things instead of staying still.

- **Difficulties communicating.** Struggling to find the right words for things, or saying the same things over and over are common symptoms of dementia. It can become difficult or tiring to engage in, and follow, a conversation, which means that people with dementia often appear to become increasingly withdrawn or quiet during social occasions.

- **Personality changes.** Mood swings, anxiety and depression are all symptoms of dementia. Coupled with problems of communication and disorientation, these symptoms can lead to reduced self confidence overall.

Getting a diagnosis

Remember: being forgetful doesn't necessarily mean you have dementia. Memory problems are anyway more likely as you get older and stress, depression and even certain vitamin deficiencies can all impact your cognitive ability.

However, if you're worried about your memory, start by visiting your GP. He or she can assess you and run various physical tests (including blood tests to make sure there is not a physical cause for your memory problems, such as a deficiency of vitamin B12), as well as mental agility tests involving questions to test your thinking, memory and orientation.

If the results of your GP's assessment indicate there may be an underlying problem, he or she may then refer you to a memory clinic where you may see a psychiatrist or neurologist for further assessment.

Here, you may be offered a CT (computerised tomography) or MRI (magnetic resonance imaging) scan. Both these tools are useful as they can identify – or rule out – conditions that have similar symptoms to dementia. Among them are a brain bleed or tumour, or a build-up of fluid inside your brain. On the other hand, the scans may show that your brain has shrunk in certain areas, which can be an indicator of dementia. An MRI scan, in particular, may show changes that have been caused by diseased blood vessels in your brain, indicating stroke or vascular dementia.

However, it's important to note that even if a CT or MRI scan shows no unexpected changes to your brain, you may still have a condition such as Alzheimer's. In the early stages of the disease, the changes to the brain can be difficult to distinguish from those we'd expect to see as a result of normal ageing.

If the results from a CT or MRI scan are still unclear (for example, if your doctors are unable to diagnose dementia or, if it is dementia, what type you have), you may be offered a SPECT (single photon emission computerised tomography) or other more specialised scan. These tests can show areas in the brain where there is a reduced amount of activity.

To make the final diagnosis, a consultant brings together medical history, as well as information gleaned from symptoms, the physical exam, the tests and any scans. The combined picture will help him or her to make the diagnosis. If that diagnosis does point to dementia, a consultant should also, by this time, be able to establish what type it is.

At this point, you may be referred for specialist help and support for your dementia; or (even with a positive diagnosis) you may be discharged back to your GP, with the option to be referred back for specialist help further down the line.

Mild cognitive impairment

Sometimes a consultant may diagnose mild cognitive impairment (MCI) rather than dementia, if the symptoms (such as memory loss) are mild or could be a sign of depression. A patient who gets a diagnosis of MCI may be discharged with a letter for their GP, asking the GP to re-refer if that patient is significantly worse after a further six to 12 months.

New diagnostic tests

At the moment, the only way the medical profession can offer a definite diagnosis of dementia is after death, during an autopsy. Scientists and researchers are constantly identifying and developing new ways to test those who are at risk, or who show early signs of cognitive impairment, in order to find a way to offer firm diagnosis during life. It may be that in the future we will be offered a combination of several tests that include scans and some or all of the options below, in order to bring forward diagnosis. Some current areas for research are:

- **Lumbar puncture.** Also known as a spinal tap, a lumbar puncture withdraws a small amount of the fluid around the spinal column. Spinal fluid is then analysed for the presence of two proteins – beta-amyloid and tau – which are present in those suffering from Alzheimer's (see the following chapter). An uncomfortable procedure, a lumbar puncture can cause side effects including headaches, back pain and bleeding around the puncture site.

- **Blood test.** Far less invasive than a lumbar puncture, a blood test can look for the presence of ten particular proteins that occur in the blood of people with mild cognitive impairment. Research shows that the presence of these proteins can predict with 87 per cent accuracy those who will go on to develop Alzheimer's within one year.[1]

- **Eye test.** People talk about the eyes being 'windows to the soul', but they are also a window to your brain: it may be possible to see changes that are happening in your brain with a simple eye test.

Researchers from Moorfields Eye Hospital in London and at Oxford University have looked at the thickness of the layer of neurons on the retina (at the back of the eye) in 33,000 people aged 40 to 69. The same cohort of people has also been asked to complete tests in memory and reasoning. Researchers have found that those people who had a thinner layer of neurons on their retina did not do as well on the cognitive tests.[2]

Other research has shown that it is possible to see deposits of beta-amyloid (a peptide, which is made up of a chain of amino acids) on the retinas of people with Alzheimer's.[3] We know that Alzheimer's causes changes in the brain that happen years before any memory symptoms. With this in mind, researchers think it might be possible to use a simple, non-invasive eye test to identify people who might be at risk of developing dementia. With early knowledge we would be able to make early interventions that could slow down the progression of the disease.

Alzheimer's and macular degeneration

Research shows that there is a link between Alzheimer's and age-related macular degeneration (AMD; a disease of the eye that causes sufferers to lose their central vision over time) – although the precise link is still unknown. Characterised by abnormal deposits, oxidative stress and inflammation, both diseases are considered to be quite similar and we know that people with Alzheimer's have an increased risk of AMD.[4] Researchers hypothesise that Alzheimer's and AMD have the same root cause, but manifest in different parts of the body. We also know that some nutrients, such as omega 3 fatty acids (see p.100) are important in the natural treatment of both conditions. Finding answers that help us understand one condition, therefore, could also help us to understand the other.

- **Sniff test.** One of the earliest areas of the brain that Alzheimer's affects is smell. One specific research study showed that those who suffered from Alzheimer's were less able to identify 12 different aromas; including apple, banana and motor oil;

than those who were not suffering from the disease. The test could identify those who had Alzheimer's with an accuracy of 86.7 per cent.[5]

- **Memory test.** The Six Item Cognitive Impairment Test (6CIT Test), refined by a British doctor[6] in response to a test already in place in the USA, screens those who are thought to be at risk of dementia. This test was developed in 1983 by regression analysis of the Blessed Information Memory Concentration Scale (BIMC) by Katzman et al in the USA. It consists of six questions that are simple, non-cultural and don't require any complex interpretation. The original test had a complex scoring system which was simplified into the 6CIT – Kingshill Version by Dr Patrick Brooke a GP and Clinical Leader in Solihull. More information is available at www.6cit.co.uk. The box below sets out the test. You'll need a partner to ask you the questions.

The Six Item Cognitive Impairment Test

This test is used to screen those individuals who are thought to be at risk of dementia. You can have a go at testing yourself, but you'll need a partner to read you the questions and note down your score for each question. At the end, add up your score to give you a total out of 28.

Before you begin, the questioner needs to find a random address (make one up or look one up on the internet – it must be something unfamiliar) with five parts (such as Mary [1] Jones [2], 32 [3] High Street [4], Essex [5], where the numbers in square brackets denote each of the five parts) and repeat it clearly to the person being tested after you've asked (and had the answer to) question 2. For all the questions the answers are spoken, not written down.

1. What year is it? Score 0 for a correct answer; 4 if the answer is incorrect.

2. What month is it? Score 0 for a correct answer; 3 if the answer is incorrect.

The questioner reads the name and address now and asks the participant to remember it.

3. **Without looking at a clock, what time is it to the nearest hour?** Score 0 for a correct answer; 3 if the answer is incorrect.

4. **Count backwards from 20 to 1.** Score 0 if there are no errors; 2 if there is one error only; or 4 for two or more errors.

5. **Recite the months of the year in reverse order.** Score 0 if there are no errors; 2 if there is one error only; or 4 for two or more errors.

6. **Tell me the name and address that I gave you earlier?** Score 0 if there are no errors; 2 if there is one error only; 4 for two; 6 for three errors; 8 for four errors; and 10 if the name and address are completely wrong.

Interpreting the score

0–7: No sign of memory problems.

8 or 9: Some evidence of memory problems; see your doctor.

10–28: High evidence of memory impairment; see your doctor to begin further investigation.

Chapter 3

What is Alzheimer's?

In the last chapter we learned that dementia is an umbrella term for up to 100 different types of disease. It's likely that the dementia disease you've most often heard of is Alzheimer's. Accounting for 50 to 75 per cent of dementia cases, Alzheimer's kills more people each year than breast and prostate cancer combined. Globally, some 30 million people are losing their memories, owing to this devastating brain disease, and every four minutes someone new is told that they have it, making it one of the world's most feared conditions – especially in the over-45s.

The progression of Alzheimer's

In the case of Alzheimer's the neurological problems – the communication between the synapses – tend to begin in the hippocampus.

Sitting inside the temporal lobes on each side of your brain, near your temples, the hippocampus is the part of your brain that forms new memories – especially new episodic memories, based on your everyday life experiences. If your hippocampus is damaged or diseased it will be harder to make these new memories and keep them, and this is why people with Alzheimer's have problems with their short-term memory – usually one of the first things they, or their loved ones, notice.

The importance of the hippocampus

Illustrating just how important the hippocampus is to memory is a famous medical case from 1933. A seven-year-old boy called HM, who had been knocked off his bicycle, started developing seizures as a result of the damage to his brain. Twenty years later, doctors removed HM's hippocampus to stop his seizures. The operation was a success – HM had no more seizures. But now, without a hippocampus, HM was unable to make new memories. In fact, he could retain new information for only 20 seconds. Of the two main types of memory – declarative (places, names, facts and events) and procedural (how to do things like tying shoelaces) – HM was left with only the second type. He could remember the long-established habits and routines he'd learned years before; but he could not remember anything new. The story of HM inspired the film *Memento*.

When you remember where you were on a certain day, and what you did and felt on that day, the information from that experience has been gathered by your senses and sent to your hippocampus for short-term storage. Over time, the memories from this part of your brain transfer into long-term storage in your cerebral cortex.

When these new memories are still fairly newly transferred and fresh in the cortex, you still use your hippocampus to retrieve them. Memories that have been in your codex for longer, and that you have thought back to many times over the years, are more embedded – it's less likely that you'll need your hippocampus to retrieve them. In what might seem a paradox, older memories, therefore, become easier to recall, because they lie in an undamaged part of the brain. Think of the Alzheimer's sufferer who may clearly remember events from their school days – in some ways appearing to have a good memory – yet struggle to remember what they had for breakfast, or even if they have had their breakfast.

Interestingly, although a person who has Alzheimer's may not be able to remember the facts or specifics about an occasion or occurrence that has happened in the recent past, he or she may be able to remember how they felt about it. This is because the course of Alzheimer's is such that the part of the brain associated with emotion – the amygdala – tends to become damaged after the hippocampus. So, a person may remember that he or she was happy or sad, but not where they were or who they were with.

As Alzheimer's spreads, different parts of the brain become affected, with different types of dementia setting in.

For example:

- As the cortex gets thinner, older memories are also lost.

- Damage to the left hemisphere (where we store our vocabulary) causes us to forget everyday words.

- Damage to the temporal lobes means that we might forget a familiar face.

- Damage to the parietal lobe, which helps us judge distances in three dimensions, can make it difficult to climb stairs.

- Damage to the frontal lobes can cause problems with decision-making, planning and organising. This kind of damage can mean that a task with a sequence of steps, such as following a new recipe, can become a challenge.

As damage in the brain spreads from the hippocampus into other areas, there is a typical progression of symptoms. First, there's loss of short term memory, then loss of language. Next comes the loss of logical thought and the ability to solve problems, followed by a change in emotions and moods. Later on, the senses become affected – causing changes in the way we perceive smell, or see and hear things, and this can lead to hallucinations. Eventually, our oldest memories disappear and then, towards the end of the disease, we lose our balance and co-ordination. At the very end of the process, the part of the brain that controls breathing and the heart shuts down. This frightening trajectory is slow and steady and lasts an average of eight to ten years. However, it is possible to live with Alzheimer's for up to 20 years.

The causes of Alzheimer's

When your brain is healthy, your thoughts and emotions travel between billions of neurons via the synapses (or junctions) that connect them. In a person who suffers from Alzheimer's, proteins (which are not the same as the protein you eat) build up on the synapses of the hippocampus, blocking the electrical signals, and disrupting the normal flow of messaging and information in your brain.

The proteins that cause damage to the synapses are called beta-amyloid proteins. As beta-amyloid proteins build up and accumulate, they form a damaging plaque. Worryingly, research shows that the build-up process shows no symptoms. In other words, the brain seems to tolerate a certain level of beta-amyloid build-up for many years before the first noticeable symptoms of Alzheimer's appear.

Because of this apparent tolerance of beta-amyloid, experts now think there must be another trigger that speeds up the damage to the synapses, taking the destruction to another level. The trigger seems to be another protein, called tau.

Tau is a protein rather like a railway track, carrying critical nutrients up and down the brain cells. It also helps to detoxify the brain of beta-amyloid plaques, preventing them from building up. The trouble seems to start when tau malfunctions. When this happens, the train tracks disintegrate, the supply of nutrients comes to a halt and beta-amyloid is spat out into the spaces between brain cells. Once there, they stick together and start to form the destructive plaques. On top of that, the tau proteins form twisted fibres known as neurofibrillary tangles. These also kill off brain cells. This destructive process can take 15 years from the time it starts to the first appearance of symptoms.

Current research is focusing on ways to tame or flush out the beta-amyloid and tau proteins that cause the plaques and tangles responsible for Alzheimer's.

The role of inflammation

As the brain becomes more diseased, it also develops inflammation, which encourages the formation of still further beta-amyloid protein plaques. This, in turn, ages the neurons, speeding up the usual age-related decline of cognitive function. Scientists used to think that this inflammation was a consequence of having Alzheimer's; but more recent research suggests that it is actually part of the disease process. If this is the case, then controlling the inflammation could be one way to treat Alzheimer's in the future.

Investigating the role of inflammation

Research shows that, among others, two inflammatory substances (IL-12 and IL-23) are present in the spinal fluid of people with Alzheimer's. Using mice bred to have the disease, researchers have blocked these two substances from reaching the brain. They found that in older Alzheimer's mice, with lots of protein plaque build-up, blocking these inflammatory substances reduced the beta-amyloid plaques and reversed the mice's cognitive decline. In younger Alzheimer's mice, it prevented the build-up of the plaque altogether.[7]

Furthermore, research carried out in 2016 has added to the evidence that inflammation may be a trigger for the disease, with scientists suggesting that blocking a receptor in the brain that regulates inflammation could help reduce changes in memory.[8] As the Alzheimer's Society in the UK says, 'This study adds to evidence that inflammation in the brain is involved in the development of the disease and suggests that by reducing this inflammation, progression of the disease may be halted.'

The role of oxidative stress

Research suggests that, as well as inflammation, oxidative stress is an important factor in the initiation and progression of Alzheimer's.[9]

Oxidative stress is what happens when your body has to cope with the damaging effects of substances called free radicals. These are natural by-products that your body produces as the result of certain bodily processes, such as breathing, but also as a consequence of such things as pollution, smoking, eating fried or barbecued food, and absorbing UV rays from the sun. Free radicals can damage healthy tissue anywhere in your body, including in your brain. The higher the levels of oxidative stress in your body, the more cell damage occurs.

Antioxidants provide natural protection from the harmful effects of free radicals, neutralising them. Foods rich in vitamins C, E and beta-carotene (the plant form of vitamin A) all have antioxidant properties, as do foods rich in the minerals selenium and zinc.

Some important plant chemicals are also antioxidants. For example lycopene (found in tomatoes), bioflavonoids (found in citrus fruits), and proanthocyanins (found in berries and grapes). The more antioxidants you have in your system, the less oxidative stress your body suffers.

The role of insulin resistance

Research shows that people with type 2 diabetes have about a 50 to 60 per cent increased risk of developing Alzheimer's. In one study participants were asked to follow one of two different diets. The first diet was packed with high-GI (Glycemic Index) foods, which release sugar quickly into the blood stream. The second was a diet rich in low-GI foods, which release sugar slowly and steadily. It took just four weeks for those on the high-GI diet to develop higher levels of insulin in their system (higher insulin is a risk factor for diabetes) and, in the same time, they developed significantly higher levels of the beta-amyloid proteins that cause damaging plaque build-up in the brains of people with Alzheimer's.[10] The research, therefore, points to a link between insulin levels and the causes of cognitive impairment.

Some other interesting research has looked at the effects of insulin on the human brain within a few hours of death. Brain activity continues for a number of hours once we have died and, knowing this, researchers soaked the brains of two groups of people (those who had had Alzheimer's and those who had not) in insulin. The brains of those who had not had Alzheimer's actively responded to the insulin. But in those who had had Alzheimer's, there was no such activity, particularly in the hippocampus.[11]

This research tells us that glucose uptake is impaired in the brain of someone with Alzheimer's. In effect, then, while the sugar – or energy – that the brain needs to function is there, the brain can't access it. We call this Brain Insulin Resistance.

A different route

Because the development of Alzheimer's follows a typical pattern, the sequence of symptoms helps doctors to diagnose the condition.

However, there's an important point here – the route is typical, but not fundamental; Alzheimer's can also show atypical symptoms. Atypical types of the disease are rare in older people – affecting only around 5 per cent of over 65s; 30 per cent of all typical cases are in under 65s.

So, what happens if the damage starts in another part of the brain? In this case, it can take longer to get a diagnosis. For example, damage to the part of your brain that controls vision might mean that the first symptom you show is a problem with your eyesight.

This is what happens with one rare form of Alzheimer's called posterior cortical atrophy (PCA). The early damage is mainly to the occipital lobes and parts of the parietal lobes, which help to process visual information and deal with spatial awareness. The early symptoms of PCA are often problems with identifying objects or with reading, even when the eyes themselves are healthy. Someone with PCA may also struggle to judge distances going down stairs or parking the car. Or they may seem uncoordinated, for example when dressing. However, the memory is likely to remain intact at first, which makes it unlikely that Alzheimer's will be the initial diagnosis that occurs to a doctor.

Early onset Alzheimer's

Early onset Alzheimer's, including the example of atypical Alzheimer's above, is rare. However, some types (though fewer than 1 in 1,000 cases) have a genetic pattern – the disease is passed from one generation to the next. There are three key genes involved in inherited Alzheimer's: the beta-amyloid precursor protein gene (APP) and two presenilin genes (PSEN1 and PSEN2). People with any of these extremely rare mutations tend to develop the disease while they are in their 30s or 40s. I will look at genes in more detail in Chapter 4.

Overall, then, as far as we know there is no single cause for Alzheimer's. However, clinical trials and medical interventions tend to focus on just one theory about the disease. In order to prevent and slow down its progression, though, we need to address as many of the possible causes as we can. That is why I believe the nutritional and lifestyle approach can be so helpful – through diet and exercise, we can try to target several different causes at the same time.

The big question

While much of the research into how to treat Alzheimer's looks at using pharmaceutical drugs to clear the beta-amyloid build-up in the brain, I think it's more helpful to ask why the beta-amyloid is building up in the first place. If we can answer that question, and then take steps to prevent the build-up occurring, we wouldn't need the medication to clear it at all.

One line of thinking is that the body produces beta-amyloid as a protective response to something else that's going on physiologically. It could, for example, be a response to inflammation, infection or oxidative stress. Or, it could be a response to exposure to environmental toxins, such as heavy metals, binding to them to help clear them from the body.

Research from Harvard University suggests that beta-amyloid, often seen as the 'baddy', is an immune-system response to something like a bacterial invasion.[12] If that is the case, then a drug therapy focused on getting rid of beta-amyloid could be counterproductive, because it's just treating the symptom and the beta-amyloid will continue to build up while the infection is still present. Stimulating the immune system – treating the cause and ridding the body of infection – would be a far more effective strategy.

The Harvard research team suggests that Alzheimer's is triggered by a normal immune response that has become overactive in response to an infection. Animal studies have shown them that beta-amyloid proteins surround and cage in bacteria in order to kill them. This tells us that the clumping effect of beta-amyloid proteins that we see in Alzheimer's is a perfectly appropriate action in response to an infection (more recent research has the same Harvard team calling beta-amyloid 'the natural antibiotic'[13]), but problematic – causing Alzheimer's – when the infection itself isn't treated.

Other research has looked at how the brain tissue in people with Alzheimer's is better able to limit the growth of the yeast *Candida* in culture, than the tissue from a healthy brain. The higher the level of beta-amyloid in the samples, the higher the brain tissue's ability to suppress the growth of the yeast.[14]

It makes sense, then, that if we fail to treat an underlying infection, the body can produce high levels of beta-amyloid that can, in turn, accumulate in the brain and clump together leading to the characteristic traits of Alzheimer's.

Interestingly, researchers in Spain have looked at the brains of people with and without Alzheimer's and found yeasts and moulds in the grey matter and blood vessels in the brains of people with Alzheimer's, but not in those without the disease. All the fungi were common ones that can live harmlessly on our skin and rarely infect us.[15]

If this is the case, then the focus of research into Alzheimer's and how to prevent or treat it needs to look at improving immune function, testing for infection, and reinstating good health, rather than just trying to find the magic bullet drug that is going to wipe out the beta-amyloid proteins.

Chapter 4

Are you at risk?

If you are worried you could be at risk of developing dementia or Alzheimer's, then you are not alone. Research shows that it is the condition most feared in the over 45s, especially if you are among the one in four people over the age of 55 who already have (or have had) a close relative with Alzheimer's or another form of dementia. However, the good news is that neither getting older, nor having a relative with Alzheimer's means that you will certainly suffer with it, too. Even when you have factors in your life that increase your risk of developing the disease, there are often steps you can take to reduce your likelihood of developing it. With that in mind, this chapter focuses on the risk factors for dementia, and what you can do about them.

Age

Age is the biggest known risk factor for Alzheimer's and dementia. While 1 in 20 people with Alzheimer's develops it under the age of 65, 1 in 14 of all people over 65, and 1 in 6 over the age of 80 will be affected. That shows just how common the problem is as we get older. But what makes some older people develop the disease while others do not?

Luck may have something to do with it – but lifestyle can also play a part. Having high blood pressure or heart disease may increase your risk as you age, particularly for vascular dementia. However, there's plenty you can do to minimise your susceptibility to heart and circulation issues: sticking to a healthy weight and taking plenty of exercise, for example, can help to both lower your blood pressure and keep your heart healthy (see box, over page).

> ## Looking after your heart
>
> Being physically inactive increases your risk of heart disease and stroke by 50 per cent.[16] Simple activities, such as walking rather than taking the car to the local shops, can make a huge difference to your general health, as well as to your heart health and stroke risk. Because vascular dementia is caused by changes in the blood flow to your brain (just as is stroke), a heart-healthy lifestyle protects your brain as well as your circulation.

Then there's just the natural process of ageing, which can also trigger Alzheimer's. Cell structure changes all over your body, including in your DNA, your nerve cells and your brain. Your body's natural repair systems weaken, your immune system changes and, if you are a woman, menopause triggers a set of hormonal changes that can themselves impact your overall wellbeing. However, my 7-step plan (in Part Two) can help to minimise the natural risks associated with the inevitability of getting older.

Gender

For most types of dementia, men and women are at equal risk. However, you are more likely to develop Alzheimer's, and suffer from it more significantly, if you are a woman, although we don't yet fully understand why (and it seems that it isn't just that statistics become skewed because women tend to live longer than men).

It seems that if we take a point in time during the progression of the disease, a woman's memory, concentration and spatial awareness will be worse than a man's at that same point in time.[17] One suggestion is that, after the menopause, lower levels of oestrogen lead to diminished cognitive function (see opposite page). Or, it could be that, traditionally, men have spent more time in work, which has given them better 'cognitive reserves' that then strengthen their brain's resistance to Alzheimer's. It also seems that women are more likely to be carriers of the gene APOE4, which is responsible for an increased risk of developing Alzheimer's.

Oestrogen, menopause and dementia

Studies show that if a woman has her ovaries removed (in order to reduce her risk of developing certain cancers), she has a greater risk of experiencing problems with her memory and other cognitive functions. Dr Gillian Einstein, of Toronto University, Canada, found that women who had had their ovaries removed did worse in word recall and logical memory tests compared with women whose reproductive systems were intact.[18] She observed that this decline in cognitive function continued for up to eight years after the ovarian surgery.

A lot of women worry about becoming more forgetful around the menopause – concerned that this may be the start of something more serious. In my clinic, many menopausal women talk about 'brain fog'. Typically, they will say that they go upstairs and can't remember what they went up for; they read a page in a book or magazine and realise they can't remember any of it; or they are suddenly unable to say the 'right' word in a sentence, finding themselves searching frantically as if they have 'lost' the word.

These memory glitches happen because we have oestrogen receptors all over our body, including in our brains. As oestrogen levels decline, so does brain function, affecting how clearly one thinks, along with memory and the ability to focus and concentrate.

But the good news is that you don't need to worry too much, because we know that brain fog and changes in memory actually equalise and return to premenopausal levels once you are past the menopause.[19] It's the hormonal fluctuations in the perimenopausal phase (when you are approaching your very last period) that cause the cognitive malfunction. Once you haven't had a period for a full year (if your menopause happens after you've turned 50; but two years if you are younger than 50), your cognitive function will start to normalise again.

Interestingly, if you begin HRT before you have your last period, there is a beneficial effect on memory and cognitive performance. However, if you start it after your last period it has a detrimental, negative effect on cognitive performance.

In my book *Natural Solutions to the Menopause,* I wrote about how, after a natural menopause when hormone levels fall off slowly, taking HRT can increase a woman's risk of breast cancer. But this risk does not apply to women who go through an early menopause when the medication is genuinely replacing the hormones that should be there, but aren't. It may be that, for a woman who suffers early menopause or enforced menopause following the removal of her ovaries, hormone replacement until she reaches the age at which she would have gone through a natural menopause (at around the age of 50) would help to stop the cognitive decline.

It is also interesting to note that, while women are at greater risk of Alzheimer's than men, research has shown that men have a higher risk of mild cognitive impairment (the stage between normal ageing and Alzheimer's). One theory is that many men die earlier than women from other causes and only the toughest men survive.[20]

Overall, though, Alzheimer's is now the biggest killer of women in the UK (causing three times more deaths than breast cancer and overtaking heart disease) and the third biggest killer for men. So, whatever your gender, finding ways to prevent the onset of dementia is essential for prolonging life.

Ethnicity

Certain ethnicities seem to have a higher risk of dementia, as well as a higher risk of other conditions that are linked to dementia. For example, people from southern Asia seem to be at greater risk of vascular dementia than white Europeans, probably because they are at greater risk of stroke, heart disease and type 2 diabetes, all of which we know raises the vascular dementia risk. Similarly, people of African or Afro-Caribbean origin are at greater risk of type 2 diabetes and stroke, and again in turn, dementia. It's important to remember that ethnicity is not just about your genes, but also about your culture and lifestyle. Genes will influence your risk, but so will your diet and fitness and whether or not you smoke.

Genes

You may worry that dementia – especially Alzheimer's – is in your genes. Some genes do directly cause early onset Alzheimer's, affecting those people aged between 30 and 60. Overall, though, according to the Alzheimer's Association in the USA, genetics are responsible for less than 5 per cent of all Alzheimer's cases.

Interestingly, about 20 genes have been identified as genes that *increase* the risk of developing Alzheimer's, although they do not *cause* it. This difference is important: some people carry the gene that increases their risk, yet they do not develop the disease; others develop the disease, but do not carry any genes that would have increased their risk. It's important to remember that if you have a strong family history of dementia, or you carry one of the genes that could increase your risk of developing it, you are certainly not guaranteed to get it – this is because of something we call epigenetics (see below).

Epigenetics – switching genes on and off

Years ago we believed that if a gene existed in a person's make-up, its effects were inevitable. Now, we understand that all sorts of things can influence whether or not a gene is 'expressed'; whether it is switched on or off. Diet and lifestyle, exposure to toxins, your environment and even whether or not your parents or grandparents smoked or ate healthily during their own lives can determine whether or not a certain gene in your body becomes active – even though none of these environmental factors change the genetic code itself. Living healthily is not just protecting your life, but the lives of your children and your children's children – and beyond – too.

Epigenetics, then, is the scientific study that looks at how your environment can influence your genes: you have a set of genes that are fixed (they are what they are), but you can influence whether or not they are activated through your environment and lifestyle decisions.

A simple way to illustrate how this works would be to think of a man who inherits the gene for being tall from one or both of his parents. However, he grows up in a place where food is scarce, and he is malnourished. As a result his growth becomes stunted and he doesn't reach his full height potential. His environment had an impact on the expression of his gene for 'tallness'. Similarly, whether or not we develop a disease can be influenced by our environment. Take two men who drink and smoke the same amount throughout their adulthood. However, one man does no exercise and eats lots of saturated fats, salt and other unhealthy foods, and the other exercises regularly and eats plenty of fresh fruit and vegetables and healthy protein. Both men carry the same gene that makes them susceptible by heredity to heart disease. The first man, whose diet and lifestyle were poor, dies of a heart attack at the age of 45; the other is still going strong at the age of 80. This isn't to say that you can always undo unhealthy choices by balancing them with healthy ones – it's merely a way to illustrate that inherent susceptibility is one factor that determines our risk for disease, and we can sometimes influence that susceptibility through lifestyle choices.

Some genes are fixed, for example your blood group is determined from birth and so is sex selection. But in some animals the environment makes a huge difference in sex selection. When crocodile eggs are laid in the sand, the temperature of the sand determines whether it is going to be a female or male. Low and high temperatures result in females and middle temperatures produce males.

The Centres for Disease Control and Prevention (CDC) Office of Genetics and Disease Prevention in the USA have produced a Gene-Environment Interaction Fact Sheet[21] that states: 'Virtually all human diseases result from the interaction of genetic susceptibility factors and modifiable environmental factors, broadly defined to include infectious, chemical, physical, nutritional, and behavioural factors.' And that: 'Genetic variations do not cause disease but rather influence a person's susceptibility to environmental factors.'

So we have:

Genes + Environment = Genetic Expression (which can mean disease or health)

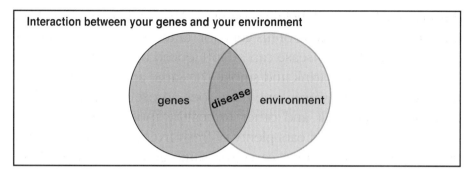

Interaction between your genes and your environment

genes   *disease*   environment

Looking at your environment and using it to minimise your risk of developing dementia or Alzheimer's forms a huge part of my 7-step plan in Part Two.

The gene that has the strongest influence on risk of Alzheimer's is apolipoprotein E (APOE), which is located on chromosome 19 (there are other genes associated with Alzheimer's, but none as significant as APOE). APOE carries cholesterol, supporting the transport of lipids (blood fats) around your body. It helps repair injuries in your brain and also helps to transport and clear beta-amyloid deposits. However, if you inherit a faulty version of APOE, your risk of Alzheimer's is increased. A simple blood test can tell you if you carry the APOE gene and even analyse your risk of developing Alzheimer's – but it can't tell you if you will definitely develop the condition. (If you want to do the test you can contact my clinic to organise it. See Resources, p.172)

The blood test looks at three types of APOE gene. These are known as E2, E3 and E4. If you inherit two lots of E3 (one from each of your parents) you have an average risk – a 50:50 risk – of developing Alzheimer's at some point in your life. To put this into context, about 60 per cent of the population has a 'double dose' of the APOE E3 gene and is at average risk. Up to half of this group will develop Alzheimer's by their late 80s.

Conversely, the APOE E2 form of the gene is mildly protective against Alzheimer's: people with it are slightly less likely to develop the disease. In the general population, 11 per cent has one copy of APOE E2 together with a copy of APOE E3, and 1 in 200 people (0.5 per cent) has two copies of APOE E2. If you inherit two lots of E2, or one E2 and one E3, you are 40 per cent less likely than average to develop Alzheimer's.

The APOE E4 gene increases your risk. If you have one E2 and one E4 you are 2.6 times more likely than average to develop Alzheimer's. With one E3 and one E4 you are 3.2 times more likely to develop it. The worst-case scenario, though, is to inherit two lots of E4, one from each of your parents: this makes you 14.9 times more likely to develop Alzheimer's. APOE E4 has also been linked to an increased risk of vascular dementia.

Risk of Alzheimer's and the APOE gene

Genotype	E2/E2	E2/E3	E2/E4	E3/E3	E3/E4	E4/E4
Disease Risk	40% less likely	40% less likely	2.6 times more likely	Average Risk	3.2 times more likely	14.9 times more likely

But to be really clear, these statistics are referring only to your risk. Remember: there are people who have Alzheimer's who do not have the genes that increase the risk, and there are those who have the genes that increase the risk, but never get Alzheimer's itself. The most important message you can take away is that your lifestyle choices can have a huge impact on your risk, regardless of your genes.

Head injuries

About one in five professional boxers will, later in life, develop a form of dementia known as chronic traumatic encephalopathy. This condition is thought to be caused by protein deposits forming in the brain after a head injury. But you don't have to be a boxer, of course, to get it: any severe blow to your head, especially if you are knocked out, seems to increase your risk of Alzheimer's later in life, probably because it kills or damages brain cells. It may also increase inflammation in the brain – another possible risk factor for the disease. Of course, the risk is higher if you carry the APOE4 gene and experience a head injury.

Type 2 diabetes

Usually starting in mid-life, type 2 diabetes occurs when your body struggles to cope with sugar (glucose), when it has processed it normally up until that point.

Normally, when your blood sugar level rises after eating food, cells from your pancreas receive a message telling them to release the hormone insulin which helps to keep your blood sugar level from getting too high or too low. Insulin's job is to turn the sugar, or glucose, into energy by sending it to cells all around your body where it can be used as fuel. In type 2 diabetes this chemical messenger isn't working properly – your pancreas is still producing insulin, but your insulin receptors are "insulin resistant", failing to respond to it - and this means the sugar (glucose) cannot be moved out of your blood into your cells in the normal way, resulting in a high level of blood sugar.

You are 50 to 65 per cent more likely than average to go on to develop Alzheimer's in later life if you have type 2 diabetes and research shows that many type 2 diabetics have the same kind of beta-amyloid deposits in their pancreas that are found in the brain of a person with Alzheimer's. Insulin resistance has now been so closely linked to an increased risk of Alzheimer's that some people now refer to Alzheimer's as type 3 diabetes.

The sugar connection

Scientists at Washington University School of Medicine in St Louis have shown that high levels of glucose in the blood can rapidly increase levels of beta-amyloid proteins, the key component of the plaques that build up in the brains of people with Alzheimer's. People with type 2 diabetes can't control the levels of glucose in their blood, which can spike after meals.

To understand how elevated blood sugar might affect Alzheimer's disease risk, the St Louis researchers infused glucose into the bloodstreams of mice bred to develop an Alzheimer's-like condition. In young mice without beta-amyloid plaques in their brains, doubling glucose levels in the blood increased beta-amyloid levels in the brain by 20 per cent.

When the scientists repeated the experiment in older mice that already had brain plaques, beta-amyloid levels rose by 40 per cent.[22] The researchers showed that spikes in blood glucose increased the activity of neurons in the brain, which promoted the production of beta-amyloid.

The role of sugar in the understanding of dementia is so significant I've dedicated a whole chapter to it in Part Two (see pp.88–98).

Cardiovascular disease

Your risk of both Alzheimer's and vascular dementia is thought to be double the average for your age if you have heart disease. Your brain depends on a healthy supply of blood to keep it well-nourished and fully functioning – and every heartbeat pumps about 20 to 25 per cent of your blood to your head, where your brain cells use at least 20 per cent of the food and oxygen that your blood carries. If there is damage – for example, as a result of high blood pressure or atherosclerosis (where your blood vessels get clogged) – to your blood vessels, your brain cannot get all the nourishment it needs. Studies suggest that plaques and tangles are more likely to cause Alzheimer's symptoms if strokes or damage to the brain's blood vessels are also present.

Hearing loss

A study at Johns Hopkins School of Medicine in Baltimore, USA, monitored 639 people aged 36 to 90 over a period of 18 years. None of the subjects had any problems with memory or any cognitive impairment at the start of the study. The researchers found that those who had mild, moderate and severe hearing loss had – respectively – two times, three times and five times increased risk of developing dementia, compared with those whose hearing was normal. Scientists believe that hearing loss increases the risk of dementia because, if you struggle to hear, the process of converting sounds into words, and then words into sense, requires extra cognitive effort. The theory is that the brain becomes so tired that it loses its effective processing power.[23] Evidence in the Johns Hopkins study compounds this theory:

the study found that the worse the hearing loss, the greater the risk of dementia, irrespective of age, diabetes and high blood pressure.

In addition, the Johns Hopkins researchers speculated that as hearing loss often makes people feel socially isolated, those who find it hard to hear are more likely to withdraw – another known risk factor for cognitive impairment. Similar findings came out of a study at Cardiff University, Wales, which monitored the physical and cognitive health of 1,984 adults over the course of 16 years. These researchers suggested that the loss of low-frequency sounds could be an early warning sign of vascular problems all over the body, leading not only to hearing loss, but also an increased risk of heart attacks, stroke and dementia. They go on to say that there could be a pathological link between hearing loss and dementia – that is a genetic or environmental factor; or, hearing loss could lead to dementia,[24] or even the other way round, with the early stages of dementia having an effect on the auditory system.

Other risk factors

Other conditions linked to an increased risk of dementia include depression, Parkinson's, multiple sclerosis, HIV, chronic kidney disease, anxiety and sleep apnoea (where breathing stops for a few seconds or minutes when you're asleep) – but, in many cases, we need more research to show how these links (if they exist) work; that is, what causes what.

Gum disease

Known medically as periodontitis, gum disease has been found to be linked to a six-fold increase in the rate of cognitive decline in people in the early stages of Alzheimer's.[25] This rate could accelerate further as the disease progresses, because people with Alzheimer's may not be able to look after their dental health.

Furthermore, research has found that people with higher levels of the antibodies for gum disease are also likely to have increased inflammatory markers in the body. We saw in Chapter 3 how inflammation is now thought to be one of the causes of Alzheimer's.

This means, of course, that if you can make sure that your gums are healthy, controlling inflammation in your dental health, you'll help to reduce your risk of developing dementia.

Professor Clive Holmes, senior research author at the University of Southampton, UK, has said that the results from his study 'build on previous work we have done showing how chronic inflammatory conditions have a detrimental effect on disease progression in people with Alzheimer's disease. Our study was small and lasted for six months, so further trials need to be carried out to develop these results. However, if there is a direct relationship between periodontitis and cognitive decline, as this current study suggests, then treatment of gum disease might be a possible treatment option for Alzheimer's.'

Proton Pump Inhibitors (PPIs)

PPIs are a medication to help reduce acid reflux, and they are now thought to increase the risk of developing dementia by 44 per cent.[26] Current research, which has investigated the connection between PPIs and Alzheimer's in mice, suggests that 'the avoidance of PPI medication may prevent the development of dementia', because it appears that PPIs increase the level of beta-amyloid proteins in the brain.[27]

However, it's also possible that the PPIs can hamper the body's ability to absorb certain nutrients – particularly zinc – which are important for brain function. In studies, blood levels of zinc increased by 126 per cent when people who were not using PPIs took zinc supplements, compared with only 37 per cent for those people taking PPIs. On a normal diet without taking zinc in supplement form, PPI users have a 28 per cent lower zinc level than people not using them.[28] It's possible, then, that if you're taking PPIs you could be zinc deficient, as your body may not be able to absorb the mineral efficiently from your food. You can be tested to see if you are lacking in zinc (see Resources Page 172).

Over-the-counter medicines

A number of over-the-counter medicines include anticholinergics – you'll find them in treatments for colds, flu, heartburn and sleep problems at your local pharmacy. However, these medications block the chemical acetylcholine, which your body needs to transmit electrical impulses between nerve cells. Recent research shows that those people taking these drugs have reduced brain volume (known as brain shrinkage) and larger cavities in their brains. They also performed less well on memory tests.[29] We'll look more into the role of acetylcholine in the treatment of Alzheimer's in Chapter 5.

Lifestyle

Your lifestyle choices greatly affect your risk of developing dementia or Alzheimer's. Studies show that people with the healthiest habits in mid-life have a lower risk of dementia later on, especially if they do three or more of the following: take regular exercise, avoid smoking, drink only in moderation, and maintain a healthy weight and diet. All of these, and more, are covered in detail in Part Two of the book but, in the meantime, check your own risk by asking yourself the following:

- **How healthy is your diet?** Too much salt, sugar and saturated fat are linked to an increased risk of dementia, as is a deficiency in certain nutrients.

- **How much alcohol do you drink?** Some experts used to think that low to moderate levels of alcohol consumption (a few units each week) could actually reduce your risk of dementia – mainly because it was also thought to help to keep the heart healthy. However, that idea is now going out of fashion.

- **How fit are you?** Physical inactivity is one of the strongest lifestyle risk factors for developing dementia. In one study, memory improved after only four weeks (one hour a day, three days a week, over four weeks) of an exercise routine that combined an aerobic workout, strength training and stretching.[30]

- **How stressed do you feel?** It is well-documented that feeling under stress has a negative impact on your memory and concentration.

- **How well do you sleep?** During deep sleep, beta-amyloid proteins are cleared from the brain – which, of course, reduces the risk of plaque build-up.

- **Do you smoke?** Smoking damages the blood vessels in the brain as well as those in the heart and lungs. According to a World Health Organisation (WHO) report published in 2014, smokers are at 45 per cent increased risk of dementia, particularly Alzheimer's, in later life. The report concludes that 14 per cent of Alzheimer's cases in the world may be the consequence of smoking.

Toxoplasmosis

The *toxoplasma gondii* parasite causes a food-borne infection called toxoplasmosis. Cats are the reproductive hosts of this parasite, which means they carry it in their digestive system. We become at risk of catching the infection when we clean out their litter trays – coming into contact with cat faeces – but there are other routes of infection, too. For example, eating raw or undercooked meat (which could carry the parasite, which has not been killed off during cooking), chopping then eating other raw foods that have been cross-contaminated (for example, by using the same, unwashed knife or chopping board) by infected by raw, contaminated meat, or drinking contaminated water. Eating unwashed fruit and vegetables that have been picked from the garden (where cats may defecate), and failing to wash hands after gardening are other possible sources.

Before you are too alarmed, it's important to know that in most people the parasite causes no harm at all. However, it can have devastating effects on an unborn baby if the pregnant mother becomes infected and it is now thought that toxoplasmosis could have profound effects on brain function and memory in older people, and could even be a cause of Alzheimer's.

The Food Standards Agency estimates that up to 350,000 people in the UK every year become infected with *toxoplasma gondii*, while the Centres for Disease Control in the USA estimates that more than 60 million Americans may be infected with it. A blood test can reveal whether or not you have antibodies in your system that have killed off a toxoplasmosis infection in your body in the past, making you immune to future infection.[31] It's thought that about 30 per cent of the population in the UK test positive for the toxoplasmosis antibodies.

However, even once your body has successfully fought off the infection, the parasite becomes dormant in your body (called latent toxoplasmosis). Researchers now wonder if, because the parasite targets the central nervous system and the brain, the dormant parasite could affect cognitive function and particularly memory in older people. Comparing people over the age of 65 who had the toxoplasma antibody to those who didn't, researchers found that those who had the antibody performed less well by about 35 per cent on tests involving short-term (working) memory.[32]

More recent research confirms this finding. In more than 4,000 people aged 60 or over, those with the toxoplasma antibody scored significantly lower on the tests for short-term memory.[33] There was no effect on long-term memory.

Preventing toxoplasmosis

You can reduce your risk of contracting the toxoplasmosis parasite by:

- Not eating raw or undercooked meat – lamb and pork are the worst culprits.

- Making sure you wash knives, utensils and chopping boards after cutting up raw meat.

- Washing your hands before and after handling food.

- Wearing gloves while gardening.

- Not having direct contact with cat faeces in a litter tray, and always wearing gloves when cleaning out a litter tray.

- Washing fruit and vegetables before eating them, especially if they have come straight from the garden.

- Not feeding your cat raw meat in case the meat is infected.

- Keeping children's sandpits covered to stop cats using them as litter trays.

• Drinking bottled water when you're unsure whether other sources of drinking water may have been contaminated.

The Centres for Disease Control (CDC) in the USA also makes recommendations about cooking temperatures for meat and poultry and says not to sample the food until it has been properly cooked. For red meat they recommend cooking to an internal temperature of at least 63°C (145°F) in the thickest part of the meat; and to at least 74°C (165°F) for poultry. Allow all meat to rest for at least three minutes before you start carving and eating, so that the internal heat of the resting meat continues to kill off any parasites or other pathogens.

When it feels like dementia, but isn't

There are some diseases, environmental factors or even medications that give symptoms very similar to dementia, but are not actually dementia itself or even risk factors for this disease. It's worth knowing about these in order to ensure you rule them out when assessing your risk and during the diagnostic process.

Statin medication

Millions of people take statin medication to reduce their cholesterol levels. However, cholesterol is important for brain function as it aids the transmission of signals between brain cells. In fact, a quarter of your cholesterol is in your brain. If statin medication lowers your cholesterol too much, you could find that your cognitive function becomes impaired. Indeed, memory loss is listed as one of the side-effects of statin medication – although the effect does seem to be reversible once you stop taking the drugs. *(If you are on statins and are noticing changes in your memory, it is important to speak to your doctor before stopping the medication.)*

Urinary tract infections (UTIs)

In a younger person, a UTI manifests itself as pain on urination or a need to urinate more frequently. However, as we get older UTIs show different symptoms – notably, confusion, agitation and even aggression. These symptoms may seem like those relating to Alzheimer's. UTIs can make Alzheimer's symptoms worse, but they are not a risk factor for or cause of Alzheimer's or dementia. Symptoms of delirium and hallucinations are common with people with Alzheimer's who have a UTI.

Lyme disease

About ten years ago the singer Kris Kristofferson started to experience memory loss. Then, in 2013, he was diagnosed with Alzheimer's. After further tests, in 2016, the diagnosis was changed – in fact, he had Lyme disease.

A bacterial infection, Lyme disease is caused by an infected tick bite. Often there is a hallmark bullseye rash around the tick bite, which may be accompanied by flu-like symptoms. The infection requires early treatment with antibiotics, because without treatment it can lie unnoticed, with serious symptoms (including heart problems, chronic fatigue, inflammatory arthritis, memory problems and lack of concentration – many of which could be mistaken for Alzheimer's) appearing only years later.

Chapter 5

Drug treatments

At the time of writing, the situation with regard to Alzheimer's is that 'Alzheimer's disease is a devastating condition with no known effective treatment'[34] and 'There are no treatments to cure or halt the progression of Alzheimer's; the currently approved pharmacotherapies provide only modest and transient symptomatic benefit.'[35]

I wanted to make this clear at the start of this chapter because it puts pharmacological intervention in the treatment of Alzheimer's into context. My belief is that drugs can treat only one aspect of the disease; whereas a more integrated approach, that harnesses the benefits of, for example, a nutritious diet, regular exercise and de-stressing techniques, can help to target several of the contributing causes of the disease.

There's an additional problem, too. Oxford researchers have noted that drug therapy in the treatment of Alzheimer's is likely to be most effective when patients are in the earliest stages of the disease. However, it can take up to ten years for symptoms to show, so, by the time a person with Alzheimer's is selected for inclusion on a pharmaceutical testing programme and the drugs have passed safety tests to say they are suitable for human trial, it's likely that subjects will be too far advanced in their Alzheimer's to really see any benefit. The solution is for pharmaceutical companies and research projects to select trial subjects following a series of expensive tests to detect the earliest stages of the disease.

All that said, in order to present a comprehensive view of the Alzheimer's journey, I want to look at two of the drugs currently prescribed for those with the disease and how they work. They are acetylcholinesterase inhibitors (also known as cholinesterase inhibitors) and NMDA receptor antagonists.

Acetylcholinesterase inhibitors

With the generic name of donepezil, this drug is best known under the brand name Aricept. Similar drugs are rivastigmine and galantamine.

Acetylcholinesterase inhibitors prevent the breakdown of acetylcholine (see p.112), which is important for memory and reasoning, thus slowing down the progression of Alzheimer's – but they are not a cure for it. Common side effects of acetylcholinesterase inhibitors can include diarrhoea, nausea, vomiting, loss of appetite, muscle pain, tiredness and sleep problems.

NMDA receptor antagonists

A glutamate receptor, this drug is best known as memantine. NMDA (N-methyl-D-aspartate) blocks the effects of the excess glutamate that is released when brain cells are damaged by Alzheimer's. Side effects can include headaches, tiredness, high blood pressure, constipation and dizziness.

The power of two

Because these two drugs work on the brain and body in different ways, it seems logical that there may be a case for combining them. One study suggests that someone who is already taking an acetylcholinesterase inhibitor gains 50 per cent greater benefit by adding in memantine, compared with taking either of the drugs on their own.[36]

It's also worth saying here that there are ways in which we can use diet and nutrition to increase acetylcholine levels and improve blood-flow and the body's natural anti-inflammatories – we'll look at these in Chapter 8.

Old drugs, new purpose

While there are two drugs specifically intended to target Alzheimer's, other drugs (intended for other medical conditions) may help this and other forms of dementia, too.

Blood pressure medication

Originally developed to treat hypertension (although not very successfully), Viagra surprised researchers by working miracles for erectile dysfunction. It increases blood flow to the genitals, and researchers think that the same sort of drug might help with increasing blood flow to the brain, helping to prevent vascular dementia. Scientists at St George's Hospital, University of London, are testing a drug called tadalafil, which is similar to Viagra, looking it into its effects on memory loss.

Furthermore, a drug called losartan, which is an angiotensin-II receptor antagonist, usually prescribed to help lower blood pressure, is being trialled to see if it can reduce brain shrinkage and improve blood flow to the brain, and so improve memory in Alzheimer's patients.

Diabetes medication

We've already touched on the links between dementia and insulin (see p.35), so it makes sense that it could be possible to treat dementia with insulin sensitisers (such as metformin) intended as treatment for type 2 diabetes, aiming to improve brain function and slow the rate of cognitive decline.[37]

Antibiotics

Researchers have shown that giving mice antibiotics reduces levels of beta-amyloid in their brains. The researchers think that the antibiotics are changing the balance of the gut bacteria, which regulates immunity and the formation of amyloid.[38] However, it may be that the antibiotics are not only changing the gut flora, but also treating an underlying infection that's leading to the production of beta-amyloid in the first place.

New treatments

Of course, the world of dementia research never stands still. New treatments are constantly undergoing investigation. Here are some that researchers are looking into at the time of writing.

Immune therapy

This new approach looks at preventing the proliferation of beta-amyloid protein and breaking up existing plaques. The drugs currently under trial are solanezumab, gantenerumab, crenezumab and aducanumab. They provide an immune therapy, giving patients monoclonal antibodies that have been taken from elderly people who do not have memory problems. Scientists hypothesise that because the immune systems of elderly people without Alzheimer's have protected them against the disease, introducing anti-beta-amyloid antibodies into someone who is in the very early stages of the disease might slow cognitive decline.

Recent research into the effects of aducanumab did show a slowing of decline when people with mild Alzheimer's were given one year of monthly intravenous infusions.[39] However, this benefit came with some significant side effects, including headaches, urinary tract infections, upper respiratory tract infections, and – most worryingly – ARIA (Amyloid-related imaging abnormalities),[40] which causes the brain to swell and the blood vessels to leak. As with any drug treatment, clinicians have to make a judgement as to whether the benefits outweigh the risks. With Alzheimer's patients, clinical trials have had a very high failure rate. Most phase 2 clinical trials ending with a positive outcome do not succeed in phase 3, often due to serious adverse effects or lack of therapeutic efficacy.[41]

In November 2016 it was announced that solanezumab, which was the first drug expected to slow down dementia, had not worked in the last trial. Initial research ongoing for more than 15 years had shown that this drug might clear beta-amyloid protein. But the latest trial of 2,000 people showed no benefit for people with mild Alzheimer's and that they showed the same rate of cognitive decline as those people on the placebo treatment.

A drug still in its animal trial stages is IL-33 (Interleukin-33). This protein, made in our bodies and especially in our brain and spinal cord, is thought to activate immune cells to engulf excess beta-amyloid and reduce inflammation.[42] Alzheimer's patients characteristically have low levels of IL-33. Tests on mice genetically engineered to have memory loss, show fast, positive results. Following injections of IL-33, the animals' memories returned within seven to ten days, regardless of where in the stages of memory loss they were. Levels of beta-amyloid in the mice's blood halved within two days of having the treatment.

LMTX

This drug targets the harmful tau protein to stop it forming tangles. It is a modification of a drug called methylene blue, which was first used as an anti-malaria treatment in the 19th century. LMTX is taken as a pill and preliminary results show that people taking the drug have 38 per cent less brain shrinkage compared to a placebo. There was also an 85 per cent reduction in moving from mild to moderate Alzheimer's.[43] It is interesting that this drug initially did not show good results when it was given to Alzheimer's patients who were also taking other dementia medication; it worked better when it was taken in isolation.

Paving the way for holistic treatment

At the end of 2013, a letter was signed by a group of leading doctors from the G8 countries addressed to the then Health Secretary Jeremy Hunt and Prime Minister David Cameron urging them not to overlook the importance of diet and lifestyle factors in reducing the risk of dementia. The letter is signed by UK doctors including former Professor Clare Gerada (Chair of the Royal College of General Practitioners), Professor David Haslam (Chair of the National Obesity Forum), Simon Capewell (Professor of Clinical Epidemiology at the University of Liverpool) and Dr Aseem Malhotra (a London cardiologist), as well as doctors from other G8 countries.

The letter stated 'The nutritional aspects of dementia are being overlooked, whether in supplement form and/or diet and lifestyle in favour of drug approaches which up until now have not been very successful.'

This was highlighted again in June 2014 when former UK prime minister David Cameron was speaking at a summit of world health and finance leaders in London. The World Dementia Envoy says progress on research has been 'achingly slow' and 'a cure impossible without a shift in approach'. The UK is launching the world's biggest study group for dementia and a new £100 million research campaign. The plan is that the UK will bring forward specific proposals on patent extensions, earlier access to new drugs for patients and greater research collaboration, and facilitate high levels of investment.

The drug approach to Alzheimer's is constantly in the news, because that is where the money is. Any company that develops a successful treatment for Alzheimer's will profit enormously. Meanwhile, changes in diet and lifestyle – which really can have a positive effect – are being overlooked. But what we all need to take away from this is that these lifestyle measures are freely available and can have an enormous effect. We should, therefore, make the most of them rather than hanging on for a miracle drug.

Where self-help steps in

The remainder of this book presents seven steps, supported with evidence, that you can take yourself in order to minimise your risk or slow the onset of dementia or Alzheimer's, or, if you have already been diagnosed with Alzheimer's or dementia, do all you can to slow its progress. Without a magical pharmaceutical cure, taking an holistic approach to disease, and treating the whole body in order to treat the brain, is a practical – and often effective – approach.

The steps in Part Two are the seven most important steps I think you need to follow in order to protect your brain. How strictly you follow these steps will depend on your situation. You might have just started to notice some memory loss and want to do something about it straightaway, or you may have a strong family history of dementia or Alzheimer's and you want to prevent your own cognitive decline.

If you have already been diagnosed with Alzheimer's and are in the early stages of the disease, you need to follow the steps more strictly. I should say, though, that this brain-protection plan is not going to work as well for someone over the age of 75 who has advanced Alzheimer's and especially if that person is taking medication as it would be for someone younger, in the early stages of the disease. Please keep an open mind and remain hopeful, but realistic with regard to your own situation. The seven steps are:

1. Your diet
2. Nutritional supplements
3. Exercise
4. Stress and sleep
5. Your environment
6. Brain training
7. Testing, testing…

PART TWO

YOUR 7-STEP BRAIN PROTECTION PLAN

Chapter 6

Step 1 (a): Your diet

As I am a nutritionist, the aspect of self-care in preventing Alzheimer's and dementia I am most interested in is, of course, diet – and I believe that what you eat can have a huge impact on the health of your brain. So let's look at what we know so far about the importance of nutrition.

The Mediterranean diet

The Mediterranean diet is routinely held up as the best example of how we should all be eating. But what is it exactly? Of course we know it takes its name from the traditional eating habits of people living in Italy, France, Greece and Spain – but there is one little problem: the food varies between these different regions, so there's really no consensus on exactly what elements of the so-called Mediterranean diet are, in fact, the active parts of the nutritional magic. The generic Mediterranean diet is, for example, a diet rich in plant-based foods, such as vegetables, fruits, whole grains, legumes, nuts and seeds; herbs and spices (rather than salt), cold-pressed 'virgin' oil (such as extra-virgin olive oil); and oily fish. Mediterranean culture places a high regard on the sociability of eating – the Italians, Greeks and Spanish tend to eat with family and friends rather than in front of the TV. (They also tend to supplement their diet with a healthy lifestyle – for example, having a good amount of exercise through activity that is naturally built in to their lives.)

Sticking well to this way of eating has been found to reduce the risk of mild cognitive impairment (MCI) by 28 per cent, and to reduce, by 48 per cent, the risk of MCI progressing to Alzheimer's. The Mediterranean diet, then, appears to provide us with an achievable and sustainable way to maintain a healthy memory.[44]

The MIND diet

The Mediterranean diet is clearly a good one to follow but, in a comparison of diets and their effects on Alzheimer's, researchers looking at the Mediterranean diet, the DASH diet (DASH is an acronym for Dietary Approaches to Stop Hypertension and again highlights the link between high blood pressure and dementia) and the MIND diet (which is the Mediterranean-DASH Intervention for Neurodegenerative Delay) found that if people adhered strictly to any of the three diets the nutritional benefits could reduce the risk of Alzheimer's. The MIND diet presented a 53 per cent lowered risk when subjects adhered to it closely, but even those who followed it only moderately had a 35 per cent lowered risk.[45]

Developed by Rush University Medical Centre, the MIND diet advocates eating from ten 'brain healthy' food groups. These are:

- Green leafy vegetables

- Other vegetables

- Berries

- Fish

- Wine

- Olive oil

- Nuts

- Whole grains

- Poultry

- Beans

In practice, this means that every day you should have one salad, one other vegetable, three servings of whole grains, and one small glass of wine. Most days you should snack on nuts. Every other day you should eat beans. Twice a week, you should eat poultry and berries and once a week you should eat fish.

The MIND diet has separated green leafy vegetables from other vegetables in general. It suggests that in your daily salad or other vegetable servings, you should have two servings a week of green leafy vegetables, but aim for six or more servings for the greatest brain benefits. While the Mediterranean diet doesn't make a distinction between types of vegetable, the MIND diet found that green leafy veg specifically make a difference to reducing the effects of Alzheimer's. The MIND diet is also specific about cooking with olive oil and about eating fish only once a week (in contrast to the Mediterranean diet that recommends it almost every day).

In addition to the foods you should eat, the MIND diet recommends foods you should avoid, comprising the following five unhealthy food groups:

- Red meat

- Butter and margarine (although I recommend organic butter in favour of any margarine, including as a spread, but only in moderation)

- Sweets

- Cheese

- Pastries

- Fried and fast foods

Avoid eating meat

Although the MIND diet doesn't 'ban' red meat altogether, research recommends that those following the diet should, to protect brain health, eat no more than four servings a week. That's more generous than the Mediterranean diet, which restricts red meat to just one serving a week.

Other research, by Dr Dale Bredesen of the Buck Institute for Research on Ageing, suggests using meat and poultry only 'as a condiment'.[46]

The problem with meat is that it can increase copper absorption and this is thought to be one of the factors that lie at the root of Alzheimer's.[47]

So, if you are going to eat meat and/or poultry, make sure it is organic and – even more importantly – that it comes from grass-fed animals rather than those that have been corn fed, which produce meat that has a high level of omega 6 fats (see p.75).

What's missing?

It surprises me that the MIND diet makes no mention of eggs, which are a first-class source of protein and have good levels of omega 3 fats and antioxidants, all of which are important for brain health. Eggs are also rich in choline, which your brain uses to make the neurotransmitter acetylcholine (see p.112), itself so important for brain health.[48] I recommend including eggs in your diet, eating up to 14 eggs a week. And you don't need to worry about your cholesterol: studies now show that it's a myth that eggs increase cholesterol levels.[49] Do, though, choose organic eggs whenever possible.

With the broad principles of what a brain-healthy diet looks like, let's look at some of the more detailed refinements you make to your diet to protect your cognitive function.

1. Eat unrefined carbohydrates

This step is simple, healthy dietary advice. You just need to switch your refined carbohydrates (white bread, pasta and rice, for example, in which the fibre has been removed) to unrefined, 'brown' versions (which are nutritionally complete and, therefore, balanced). In other words, develop a taste for oats and brown rice. Then you have to ensure you eat little and often, adding protein (vegetable or animal) to each meal, and never allowing your sugar levels to plummet or spike – which will tempt you to snack unhealthily.

Understanding fibre

There are two forms of fibre: soluble (which dissolves in water) and insoluble (which doesn't). Insoluble fibre, which is found in whole grains and vegetables, keeps your bowels healthy; soluble fibre, found in oats and beans, has been shown to have a very useful impact on controlling blood sugar.[50] Both help to give a sense of fullness and satisfaction.

Soya and the other legumes like chickpeas and lentils contain both soluble and insoluble fibres and research has shown that soya can decrease insulin resistance.[51]

Some foods contain so much fibre in relation to their carbohydrate content that you can eat as much as you like without any risk of a high rise in blood glucose and a subsequent high release of insulin. Examples of such 'free foods' are cooked asparagus, aubergine (eggplant), beans, broccoli, Brussels sprouts, cabbage, cauliflower and kale; raw celery, fennel, lettuce, olives, peppers and tomatoes; and raw fruits, avocados, raspberries and strawberries.

A diet that includes unrefined carbohydrates rather than refined ones, is the best way to prevent or reverse the insulin resistance that has been linked to Alzheimer's and it is also the best way to ensure that you lose weight.

The reason it works is simple. When you eat, your body breaks down all carbohydrates (sugars and starches) into glucose. The faster the carbs break down, the more dramatic (and destructive) their effects on your blood-sugar levels. A rise in blood-sugar levels triggers the pancreas to release insulin. The higher the rise in blood sugar, the more insulin the pancreas releases.

If you switch from quick-burn white foods to slow-burn whole foods, you create a steady, gradual rise in your blood sugar. The body hardly has to respond at all – having to release only a small amount of insulin to deal with it.

Put another way, some carbohydrates (refined sugar, for example) are broken down very quickly, causing a rush of glucose into the blood. Others (such as brown rice) take longer to metabolise and give the body plenty of time to deal with them.

You can gauge the speed at which your body metabolises one food relative to others using its Glycaemic Index (GI) value. A fast-burn food has a high GI; a slow-burn food has a low GI. However, if all that seems too technical and time-consuming, think simply in terms of whether the carbohydrate you're choosing to eat is refined or unrefined – and choose unrefined every time. Use the table below to help you.

Unrefined foods	Refined foods
Barley	Biscuits, cakes and pastries made with white flour and sugar
Brown rice	
Buckwheat (part of rhubarb family)	Breakfast cereals with added sugar
Fruit (particularly berries, apples and pears and citrus)	Brown and white sugar
Maize	Chocolate
Millet	Fruit juice (as the fibre has been removed)
Oats	
Rye	Honey
Spelt	Instant 'quick cook' porridge oats
Vegetables	Sugar
Quinoa	Soft fizzy drinks
Wholemeal flour	Treacle
	White flour
	White rice

After a few weeks of eating unrefined carbohydrates (each time combined with a little protein; see opposite) most people feel healthier and more alert and, in all likelihood, you'll also lose weight. Remember that refined foods contain very little goodness (so many nutrients are lost in the refining process), which means that after many years of eating unhealthily you're likely to become nutrient deficient. Your body typically responds to nutrient deficiency by increasing appetite to try to get those valuable nutrients from a larger amount of food and by storing fat (because it thinks you are starving). The more refined the food you eat, the more deficient you become and the more your appetite and cravings increase… driving you to eat more refined, nutritionally-deficient food.

> ## Fruit juice
>
> It might surprise you to learn that fruit juice is a refined carbohydrate because the juicing process removes most of the fibre, which remains in the wasted pulp. This means that the natural sugars in the fruit flow into the juice without their modifying fibre. When you drink juice the sugars hit your blood stream quickly, forcing your pancreas to pump out a lot of insulin.
>
> With this in mind, limit your intake of fruit juices if you are trying to control your insulin levels. Whole fruit, with all its fibre intact, is a much better option. In fact, one large long-term study found that increasing fruit and vegetable consumption reduced the risk of diabetes, but increasing fruit juice consumption by just one serving a day gave an 18 per cent increased risk of diabetes.[52]
>
> Finally, avoid anything called 'fruit juice drink', which is likely to contain refined sugar or artificial sweeteners. If you are drinking pure juice, dilute it 50/50 with water, or opt for a smoothie (which contains the fibre from the fruit).

2. Eat protein with every meal

You can improve the low-GI effect of unrefined carbohydrates even further if you try to include protein in every meal and most snacks. So, whenever you eat an oat cake or brown rice, include some fish or egg, or a vegetable protein such as quinoa, legumes (in the form of, say, chickpea hummus), nuts (nut butters, such as almond butter, are good) or seeds. The body takes longer to process proteins than other foods, so adding protein effectively slows down the absorption of the nutrients in your food, including the carbohydrate.

3. Eat less added sugar

The debate rages about sugar and its effects on the body and mind – so much so that I've separated it out and dedicated the whole of the next chapter to looking into its significance for cognitive decline. Nonetheless, seeing as we're talking about nutrition, let's look at the basics of reducing your sugar hit now.

It is really important to try to cut down on added sugar as much as you possibly can. Sugar is one of the most refined carbohydrates available and a real enemy for anyone trying to avoid dementia and Alzheimer's.

Cutting back on sugar can be really tough at first but, once you start eating more healthily, your tastes will naturally change and your body will crave fewer sugary foods. Don't forget that there are lots of foods that have 'hidden' added sugar – that is, they contain sugar and you may not even realise it. Research shows that some people consume around 46 teaspoons of sugar every day, some of which is buried unknowingly in their food and drinks.[53] Get used to reading the labels on food, as sugar comes in many different disguises: fructose, glucose, dextrose (made from cornstarch), lactose (milk sugar), maltose, sucrose (common table sugar made from sugar cane or beet) and corn syrup (made from corn) are all types of sugar.

Manufacturers are obliged to list ingredients in a food product with the largest ingredient first, so, to avoid the word 'SUGAR' looming large, they mix in smaller amounts of the different types of sugars.

Be aware that sugar is added to savoury foods, such as tomato ketchup and canned soup, mayonnaise and salad dressing, too. A 'healthy' fruit yogurt can contain as much as eight teaspoons of added sugar. Watch out for 'healthy'-looking breakfast cereals where some can contain more sugar than a doughnut (11.1g in a small bowl of cereal compared with 8.6g in one doughnut).

Remember that having higher levels of glucose from eating too much sugary food is a risk factor for dementia, even if you don't have diabetes.[54] My advice is to avoid any products with added sugar and think more creatively about how you use typically-sugary foods. For example, try a smearing of pure fruit (sugar-free) jam on a wholegrain cracker, and look for biscuits sweetened with apple juice – both can help wean you off added sugar (a small amount of fruit juice used as a sweetener is fine compared to a glass of fruit juice). Flapjacks made sticky and sweet with mashed banana are far better for you than those laden with syrup and brown sugar.

Personally, I don't recommend a switch to artificial sweeteners in order to avoid sugar, as studies show they can confuse your body and don't help you lose weight. In fact, I believe artificial sweeteners make your body crave other foods and can actually increase your appetite and cause you to gain weight.[55]

Blood sugar and ageing

Fluctuating blood-sugar levels that cause highs of glucose and insulin make you age faster. This is all down to the 'glycation theory of ageing', which was introduced in the 1980s and occurs when glucose (sugar) gets out of control. Glycation is the process that changes your body's protein structures (such as your skin, hair, blood vessels and organs) into substances called, appropriately, AGEs (advanced glycation end-products).

Your body is 60 per cent protein. When your body's proteins react with excess sugar in your diet cells lose their elasticity; they become hardened and can stop functioning properly. It is the same process that occurs when you heat the sugary top of a crème brulée to make the caramel crust.

These AGEs can cause changes in your skin, making it less elastic and creating more wrinkles than are appropriate for your age. The hardening effect can increase your risk of heart disease (hardening of the arteries), eye problems (cataracts) and nerve damage (where circulation and feeling deteriorates). These are the exact same complications that diabetics can suffer because of poorly or uncontrolled glucose. Scientists have found that giving animals just a small amount of glucose reduces their life span by 20 per cent.[56]

We know that having high levels of AGEs is associated with a faster rate of decline in memory[57] and that even a short-term diet of junk food can have a negative effect on your memory. Feeding rats a diet high in fat and sugar caused them to have impaired memory function and brain inflammation of the hippocampal region after just one week.[58] What was really worrying was that the results were just as bad for those rats fed a healthy diet, but who were given sugar water to drink. In other words, the benefits of the healthy diet did not outweigh the negative effects of the sugar.

The comments from the researchers are interesting: 'since

modifying the levels of AGEs in the diet may be relatively easy, these preliminary results suggest a simple strategy to diminish cognitive compromise in the elderly and warrant further investigation'.[59] And 'while nutrition affects the brain at every age, it is critical as we get older and may be important in preventing cognitive decline. An elderly person with poor diet may be more likely to have problems'.[60]

Follow my recommendations below to get your blood sugar under control and bear in mind that, by reducing or eliminating the amount of added sugar in your diet (in cakes or biscuits) and also reducing refined carbohydrates like white flour, you can not only keep your brain as healthy as possible but also extend your life span and help yourself to stay looking and feeling younger for longer.

As well as making sure you are eating as healthily as possible, think about your cooking techniques. Reduce the temperatures as low as possible (for healthier cooking) and cook with water (boil, poach or steam) most of the time instead of dry-baking, barbecuing or grilling. Water prevents sugars from binding to protein molecules so helps reduce the formation of AGEs.

4. Eat little and often

It is obvious that what you eat can have a huge impact on your blood-sugar levels, but also important is the timing of when you eat. To keep blood-sugar levels stable you need to create a slow, low rise in blood sugar after a meal, so your pancreas does not have to produce large amounts of insulin to deal with a quick sugar rush, and you need to try to maintain a steady level until you eat the next meal or snack.

The trick is to eat little and often and to allow not more than three hours to pass between meals. I recommend breakfast, lunch and dinner with a mid-morning snack and a mid-afternoon snack. Don't skip breakfast. If you do, by 10 or 11am your blood sugar will have dropped so low that your body will be urging you to go for a quick fix (a cup of coffee and a biscuit, say; a chocolatey treat or a slice of cake) to boost your blood-sugar levels so there's a little fuel for your poor, addled brain.

If you leave long gaps without eating (as so many people do when they're trying to lose weight) your body will think there is a shortage of food (a famine perhaps?) and it will very cleverly slow down your metabolism, holding tightly on to your fat stores. When you then do finally eat, it will – just as cleverly – work really hard to absorb as many calories as possible from that meal because it thinks you might not eat again for a long time.

If, on the other hand, you eat little and often you tell your body that there is an abundance of food out there. This can rev up your metabolism and your body will let go of its fat stores. Indeed, research in adolescents has shown that snackers tend to be less overweight and obese and have less fat around the middle (a risk factor for heart disease, diabetes and also Alzheimer's and vascular dementia).[61]

Sugar cravings are hard to resist if your blood sugar has dropped so low (hypoglycaemia) that your body urges you to find a quick high-sugar fix. The brain needs a constant trickle of blood sugar to function. It reacts to a blood-sugar drop by either releasing stress hormones that themselves release sugar from fat stores, or creating an impossible-to-resist craving for a quick sugar fix. This has nothing to do with weak willpower, it is a strong physiological urge designed to correct your low blood-sugar levels.

The link between insulin and Alzheimer's

We used to think that the only purpose of insulin was to regulate blood sugar, but we now know that it also regulates our neurotransmitters – the brain chemicals, such as acetylcholine, that are important for learning and memory. Insulin is important for healthy neuron function, especially in those areas of the brain most affected by Alzheimer's – the hippocampus and the frontal lobe (see p.20).

Insulin also aids the growth of the blood vessels that supply the brain with oxygen and glucose, which helps to prevent the onset of vascular dementia and promotes plasticity, whereby your brain can change over your lifetime, making new connections.

Animal studies confirm the effects of insulin on cognitive function: if animals are made to become diabetic, Alzheimer's changes in the brain occur with an increase in beta-amyloid plaques.[62]

The suggestion is that, like the body, the brain can become 'insulin resistant' – unable to respond to insulin properly. Comparing the brain response to insulin in those with and without Alzheimer's, those without Alzheimer's showed active insulin signalling in response to insulin, but those with Alzheimer's showed no such activity. Researchers conclude that people with Alzheimer's have brain insulin resistance.[63]

In another study, people were asked to follow either a high-GI diet or a low-GI diet. Within just four weeks, those on the high-GI diet had higher levels of insulin and significantly higher levels of beta amyloid taken from spinal fluid compared with those on the low-GI diet.[64]

Because of these effects, I cannot stress enough how important it is that, even if you show no signs of pre-diabetes or full-blown diabetes, you eliminate or, at the very least, drastically reduce added sugar and also refined carbohydrates (such as white bread and white pasta) from your diet.

5. Eat more healthy fats

Forget switching to a tasteless low-fat diet and boost your intake of the sort of healthy fats you find in oily fish, such as salmon, nuts and seeds. These good fats are called 'essential fatty acids' because they are essential to your health. They include polyunsaturated fats, omega 6 fats and omega 3 fats, the most important of which – for brain health – are the omega 3s.

A recent study of more than 900 older people with an average age of 81 found that those who had at least one meal of seafood a week showed less cognitive decline. What was very interesting was that there was a slower rate of decline in those who carried the APOE4 gene (the high-risk gene for Alzheimer's), with weekly seafood consumption and moderate-to-high omega 3 intake from food.[65]

Omega 3s also help to overcome insulin resistance, which can cause Alzheimer's to develop, and they have a part to play in your long-term health in terms of prevention of diabetes, obesity, high blood pressure and good heart health.[66]

Fats, ageing and inflammation

Omega 3 fatty acids help to control inflammation. On the other hand, omega 6 fatty acids can increase inflammation. Research has shown that people who have a diet high in omega 6 and low in omega 3 fatty acids produce more inflammation that is linked to Alzheimer's.[67] Furthermore, DHA, which is the major omega 3 fatty acid in your brain, seems to have the most protective effect against Alzheimer's,[68] helping to prevent the beta-amyloid plaques forming.[69]

These omega 3 fats are crucial for keeping your cell walls flexible. Without an adequate supply in the diet, cell walls harden and their insulin receptors become unresponsive, encouraging insulin resistance to set in. With a diet rich in omega 3 fats, the cell walls become healthier and their insulin receptors become more sensitive, and both willing and able to take the sugar (glucose) from your blood and use it for energy.

Supermarket shelves are awash with foods – such as some milks and bread – that claim to be fortified with omega 3 fats. Bear in mind that the additional good fats in these foods can be fairly low – you'd have to eat 23 slices of enriched bread a day to get sufficient omega 3 to make a difference. It's probably easier to eat one portion of salmon, herring, sardines or mackerel (fresh, frozen or tinned).

Finally, consider how much omega 6 fat (found in vegetable oils) you're consuming. Although omega 6s are generally good for you, eaten to excess they can undo the good work of the omega 3s. Estimates show that most people consume 25 times more omega 6 fats than omega 3. However, for good health, the ratio should be closer to 1:1.[70] A simple home finger-prick blood test can tell you if you have the correct levels of omega 6 to omega 3 in your body (see Resources page 172 for advice on how to do this).

A combination of high insulin and high ratio of omega 6 to omega 3 causes your body to produce compounds that increase the destructive inflammatory response.

Overall, my advice is increase your intake of oily fish and reduce your intake of omega 6 by cutting down on polyunsaturated vegetable oils, such as sunflower and corn oil. Olive oil, which is omega 9 oil, is good to use for cooking, as long as you keep the temperature as low as possible. If you heat the oil too high, you will produce free radicals (see p.83).

Omega 3 in the vegetarian and vegan diet

The best food sources of omega 3 are oily fish (such as salmon, mackerel and sardines), which contain good levels of EPA and DHA. Omega 3 as alpha linolenic acid (ALA), is found in seeds such as flaxseeds and chia seeds. In order to convert ALA to EPA and DHA, you need good levels of certain nutrients such as zinc, magnesium and vitamin B6. You'll get even less goodness from these foods if you are stressed and/or drinking too much alcohol. Furthermore, if you're vegetarian or vegan watch your omega 6 levels – research shows that if levels of omega 6 are too high, conversion from ALA to EPA and DHA can fall by up to 50 per cent.[71] You can get some vegetarian EPA and DHA supplements, but they usually don't contain enough of these good fats to make up the difference.

There's more on supplementation and the importance of omega 3 healthy fats in Chapter 8 (Step 2 of the 7-step plan).

I mentioned the home finger prick test above (see p.159) to check your ratio of omega 6 to 3 and I would suggest that this test is particularly important if you are vegetarian or vegan, to see how much EPA and DHA you are converting from the ALA in flaxseeds for example.

Fats make ketones

As we already know, brain glucose uptake is impaired in Alzheimer's, so this means that your brain is not getting the fuel it needs to function well. However, glucose isn't the only fuel your brain can use – it can also run on natural by-products of fat-burning, called ketones. Although

Alzheimer's affects your brain's ability to use glucose, its uptake of ketones is the same in people with Alzheimer's as in those of the same age without the disease.[72]

There are two ways of helping to fuel your brain with ketones. One is to change your diet, so that your body goes into a state of ketosis – we'll look at what this is on page 85. The other is increase your body's ketone production. Your liver can convert fats into ketones, which it releases into your blood stream for your brain to use as energy, instead of glucose. The medium chain fatty acids (MCFAs), also known as medium chain triglycerides (MCTs), found in coconut oil are a good source of the right kinds of fats for ketone conversion.

Most fats are mixed with bile released from your gallbladder in order to be broken down in your digestive system. But MCTs are broken down almost immediately by enzymes in your saliva and gastric juices and then metabolised directly by your liver into ketones, which can then be transported to your brain. Research has shown that eating 40ml (11 teaspoons) of coconut oil per day has a beneficial effect on cognitive function for people with Alzheimer's.[73] Coconut oil can also increase the levels of HDL ('good' cholesterol) and reduce your waist circumference, which we know is a risk factor for Alzheimer's.[74]

Although coconut oil has previously had a bad name because it contains a high amount of saturated fat (over 90 per cent, which is higher than butter), two-thirds of this fat is in the form of MCTs. I would suggest using organic coconut oil where possible. Start with a small amount and always have it with other food. It is better to take coconut oil in the morning as it takes about three hours for the oil, once converted into ketones, to reach your brain. You could just take it by the spoonful if that suits you or mix it into porridge or even into scrambled eggs. Or, use it in cooking – because it is a saturated fat it doesn't become damaged during the heating process, which can create free radicals in polyunsaturated oils.

Finally, it is possible to buy MCT oil, which contains a more concentrated amount MCT than found in coconut oil. However, whereas coconut oil is found in nature, MCT oil is not: it is man-made, which means the fat molecules have been separated out from their natural 'habitat', which may in itself provide beneficial modifiers. You also can't use it in cooking. Given a choice, I would always choose an organic coconut oil, rather than a man-made oil.

6. Avoid unhealthy fats

Not all fats are created equal. Your brain is 70 per cent fat – so fat is important in your diet – but it has to be the right type. There are some fats that I think you should make every attempt to reduce in your diet, or even to avoid completely, in line with the advice in the MIND diet (see p.64).

Saturated fats

I think it's a really good idea to try to reduce your intake of the saturated fats you find in meat and dairy products. A high intake of saturated fats makes it more difficult for your body to absorb omega 3 fats efficiently which, in turn, leads to increased inflammation. Research shows that saturated fats induce inflammatory activity and increase insulin resistance.

The more bad fat you have in your diet, and the more fat you accumulate around the middle of your body, the more inflammation you will have, which increases your risk of dementia. This visceral tummy fat is metabolically active and adds to the inflammation process, just making things worse. Also called adipose tissue, fat around your middle functions in its own right, manufacturing and releasing different substances and producing an immune response in your body, which causes still further inflammation. In evolutionary terms, this inflammatory response allowed your fat stores to help fight infection. They produce substances called inflammatory cytokines, which pump up the immune system and urge your adrenal glands to release cortisol. However, in many people, the excess cortisol causes the body to store yet more fat, which then releases more inflammatory cytokines.

If you are concerned about saturated fats, you don't need to become vegetarian to avoid them. I don't recommend eating meat or poultry but, if you are eating them, buy meat and poultry from organic grass-fed animals, which will contain more omega 3 fats than meat from animals fed on corn (more omega 6).

Trans fats

Trans fats are the worst fats of all – avoid them. They have been linked to an increased risk of heart disease and are terrible for your general health; they will cause you to put on more weight around your middle, even if you're sticking to a low calorie diet[75] – and we know that belly fat is linked to an increased risk of Alzheimer's (see p.129).[76]

Found in many processed foods (such as cakes, biscuits and fast foods) to prolong their shelf life, trans fats might appear on labels as hydrogenated or partially hydrogenated vegetable oil. They are produced by passing hydrogen through the oil at high temperature and under pressure to chemically alter liquid oils to make them into solids. Consuming them is as unnatural to the body as if you were to consume plastic – your body doesn't know what to do with them, so they can cause all sorts of unhealthy processes to occur.

They block the absorption of the essential fatty acids, which your body needs to overcome insulin resistance (among other things), hindering any attempts you might be making to improve insulin sensitivity. They harden cells and arteries, but they can also harden your insulin receptors, making you more insulin resistant and encouraging your body to produce even higher amounts of insulin.

Studies show that avoiding trans fats can reduce your risk of diabetes by 40 per cent.[77] Recent research confirms that trans fats can distort cell membranes, are incorporated into your brain cells and alter the ability of your neurons to communicate: 'There is growing evidence for a possible role of trans fats in the development of Alzheimer's disease and cognitive decline with age.'[78]

Not only do trans fats create more inflammation in the body, in a horrific double-negative effect, they also block the production of beneficial anti-inflammatory substances.

Interestingly, a number of authorities (including those in Denmark, Switzerland, Austria, and the city of New York, USA) have banned trans fats – not only in food products but also in restaurants and fast food outlets. In the UK, officials say a ban would be too difficult to implement, so just be vigilant and read all food labels!

Cinnamon as a natural insulin sensitiser

Try sprinkling a teaspoon of cinnamon on your porridge or into herbal tea each day. It could play a role in the long-term prevention of insulin resistance.[79] Recent research using Alzheimer's diseased rats showed that cinnamon improves learning ability[80] and that it could have neuroprotective effects on the brain. However, please note that it's not a good idea to consume large amounts of cinnamon if you have a bleeding disorder or you are taking a blood thinner, such as heparin or warfarin, as it contains a substance called courmarin, which can have a blood-thinning effect.

---

7. Cut down on caffeine

If you have, by now, made the switch to unrefined carbohydrates, you will be doing the best you can to keep your blood sugar levels on an even keel. It is the energy dips and troughs and long gaps between meals that trigger your adrenal glands into action, encouraging them to pump out the stress hormones, adrenaline and cortisol, that are also harmful to your brain health. We know that Alzheimer's risk goes up with increased levels of cortisol.

It follows that if you really are serious about lessening your risk of Alzheimer's, it is very important to try to keep those adrenal glands as happy as possible. One way to do this is to cut back on caffeine. Anything containing caffeine – including coffee, tea (black, green and white), colas and chocolate – acts as a stimulant that will make your body release more of the stress hormones and cause blood-sugar levels to fluctuate. Caffeine also acts as a diuretic, so if you drink a lot, you risk losing valuable nutrients through your urine.

However, some research suggests that coffee consumption might have a protective effect against mild cognitive impairment (MCI) and dementia. So, it's more the amount of caffeine that you consume that's significant, rather than the caffeine itself. If people without any cognitive problems increase their coffee consumption, they increase their risk of developing MCI. But in moderate coffee drinkers (one to two cups per day), there is a reduced rate of MCI.[81]

Quercetin

Other interesting research suggests that, in fact, it is not the caffeine in the coffee that, in small amounts, has a protective effect on cognitive decline, but an antioxidant called quercetin,[82] which is found in coffee but also in lots of other foods. Quercetin is a flavonoid antioxidant that has anti-inflammatory effects. It can be found in green leafy vegetables, onions, tomatoes, berries and also green and black tea.

In some impressive research, giving people with early stage Alzheimer's just a quercetin-rich onion powder over four weeks has been shown to improve memory recall.[83]

My recommendation would be to be wary of coffee or any caffeinated drinks or foods if you are stressed and/or know that your blood sugar is already on a roller coaster. And, even if you can tolerate coffee, do remember that it may not be the caffeine that is having a neuroprotective effect but antioxidants within the coffee – and you can get those antioxidants in greater amounts by eating a rainbow of fruit and vegetables (the more colours you eat, the greater the array of antioxidants). I don't recommend decaffeinated coffee, because even though the caffeine is removed, other adrenal-depleting stimulants (theobromine and theophylline) are left behind.

All the colours of tea

I regularly hear people talk about green tea as being caffeine-free – but that's not true: green tea does contain caffeine. Nonetheless, green tea is healthier than traditional black tea because is less processed and is usually drunk without milk. It contains antioxidants, which are generally beneficial to your health and can help inhibit the growth of cancer cells by inducing cell death,[84] and it can help to lower cholesterol. Green tea could also help you lose weight as it has a mild fat-burning effect[85] – in the fight against dementia this is important because we know that being overweight is linked to a higher risk of brain shrinkage, one of the hallmarks of Alzheimer's.[86]

Although there has been little research into the benefits of white tea, it is less processed than green tea, and is said to contain more antioxidant polyphenol catechins, which (among other things) may be able to protect the ageing brain and reduce the incidence of dementia and Alzheimer's.[87]

I would suggest you reduce or eliminate your intake of black tea and substitute the occasional cup of green or white tea instead, adding some herbal teas such as peppermint or chamomile into the mix. Decaffeinated tea is stimulant-free, but can contain residues of the chemicals used to remove the caffeine.

Caffeine content of different drinks (per 240ml)	
Coffee, instant	66mg
Coffee, filtered	120mg
Tea, ordinary black tea	60mg
Colas	45–50mg
Tea, green	15mg
Tea, white	15mg
Cocoa	14mg
Chocolate, dark (1oz)	20mg
Chocolate, milk (1oz)	6mg
Coffee, de-caffeinated	5mg

How to avoid caffeine withdrawal

If you have been a hardened caffeine drinker, reduce your intake slowly so as to avoid suffering withdrawal symptoms. These can be unpleasant, causing headaches, flu-like symptoms, muscle cramps and fatigue. Substitute one cup a day with a decaffeinated alternative, then, when you are drinking only decaffeinated coffee or tea, gradually substitute those, one cup a day, for herbal tea or even a grain-based coffee (which is available in health food shops and contains chicory and barley, for example).

8. Increase antioxidants

We generate free radicals through the natural processes of living and breathing (including our oxygen metabolism), but we also inhale, absorb and digest them. Free radicals come from environmental pollutants, radiation, pesticides, preservatives, cigarettes and car fumes. Free radical damage has been linked to premature ageing and many of the illnesses that are connected to us getting older, including cancer, heart disease and Alzheimer's.[88] Research suggests that these free radicals can attack brain cells, causing some of the structural changes found in Alzheimer's. Your brain is particularly susceptible to free radical damage because it uses up a lot of oxygen to produce energy and is composed of fragile unsaturated fats, such as DHA, which are easily oxidised (oxidation is the process of creating free radicals in the body).

Your body (and mind) needs antioxidants to neutralise free radicals. The most powerful antioxidant nutrients are vitamins A, C and E, and flavonoids found in fruits and vegetables. Specific research into the antioxidant benefits of pomegranates shows them to have neuroprotective effects as a result of 21 different antioxidant compounds. One of these compounds is called urolithins, which acts as an anti-inflammatory and is produced in the body when gut bacteria break down the antioxidant polyphenols in the pomegranate. Polyphenols themselves can't cross the blood–brain barrier, but urolithins can. Once they are through the barrier, the urolithins can help to control beta-amyloid plaque build-up. It seems to be pomegranate juice that has the best positive effect on brain health.[89]

9. Get some beneficial bacteria

Getting your levels of beneficial bacteria (probiotics) right can actually help you lose weight and can play a major role in helping you control inflammation, which is important for your brain health.[90]

I recommend taking probiotics in supplement form, rather than as a drink or in a yogurt, to make sure the quantities you're getting are high enough to be useful and because probiotic drinks and yogurts can be loaded with sugar. There's more about probiotic supplements in Chapter 8 (Step 2).

10. Learn about fasting

I have talked about making sure your blood sugar is balanced by eating little and often. But are there benefits for your brain health if you fast or if you restrict your calories?

Animal studies have shown that mice live 30 per cent longer when they eat half the normal amount of calories – and dogs, fish and even yeasts live longer when their calories are cut. We humans would have to reduce our calories by 25–30 per cent to achieve the same effect. And even though the research on animals has been around for eight decades, it is still not clear why calorie restriction has this effect.

Some researchers think that certain genes are turned on to help fight disease if the body perceives there is famine with the aim of making the body stronger. Other research suggests calorie restriction decreases insulin levels and stops the advanced glycation end-products (see p.71).

Although the emphasis on this type of diet is reducing the calories, the aim is also to make the diet nutrient-rich, so that you are not malnourished.

The first study on humans in 2006 showed reduced signs of ageing in those who were restricting calorie intake. The men and women on the diet had reduced fasting insulin levels and lowered markers of inflammation. Furthermore, the rate at which their DNA decayed slowed down, reducing their risk of cancer.[91] So, we know that restricting calories can increase your lifespan, but what about your brain health? Previously I talked about ketones, which your brain can use as an alternative fuel if it can't use glucose efficiently. I mentioned that there are two ways of increasing ketones. One way is to use coconut oil, and the other is to change your diet so that your body produces ketones independently.

We know that if you eat a ketogenic diet which is very high in fat and low in carbohydrates (which are converted to glucose) or are starving, your body produces more ketones and goes into what is called ketosis. During ketosis, the body compensates for the lack of carbohydrate and instead converts stored fat into ketones to use as fuel.

The theory sounds perfect – but despite the media hype about alternative day, intermittent and 5:2 dieting, the evidence is just not there yet to show that fasting diets are helpful in terms of overall health. As one researcher says, 'substantial further research in humans is needed before the use of fasting as a health intervention can be recommended'[92] because most of the research has been conducted on animals.

And, even if there are benefits, which of the very many variations of fasting diet is the one that has the best health effects? On a 5:2 fasting diet, you fast on two days a week and eat normally on the other five. But, should the fast be complete calorie restriction apart from water, or is it better to have minimal calories (usually levelled at 600 a day for men and 500 a day for women)? Should the fasting days be consecutive or are they better as any two days in the week? If you follow the 5:2 fast with limited calories, is it better to have all the calories in one meal or spread them out throughout the day? Other regimes suggest alternate-day fasting, when you are fasting every other day of the week.

On non-fasting days, no matter what regime you are following, the suggestion is that you can eat as much as you like of whatever you fancy. As a nutritionist, this makes me very uncomfortable! It suggests you can eat your fill of junk food on the non-fasting days. But that cannot do you any good at all! Generally, advocates of the fasting diets recommend that you drink water during the fast day. However, many people load up on black coffee and tea or diet drinks instead. If you use caffeine to get you through, then you are going to be living on adrenaline for the fasting days, putting your body into a permanent state of stress.

Some people swear by fasting diets for weight loss – but they are not suitable for everyone. If you are diabetic or have a history of an eating disorder or have osteoporosis, then they are certainly not for you. Likewise, if you get blood sugar swings during which you feel weak, headachey, dizzy or light headed when you don't eat. I also don't think it is good for anyone suffering from chronic fatigue or a lot of stress.

To your body, fasting is a stress, because it perceives there is a shortage of food, a threat to survival; it is a matter of life or death. So, if you are already stressed or fatigued, adding a further stress to your body is severely damaging to health. If you do a lot of exercise or are training for an event, then you are potentially doing much harm to your body by restricting calories that you need to fuel your fitness.

What's the alternative?

There seems to be a much better way to get the beneficial effects of fasting without actually restricting your calorie intake. Your body has a process called autophagy. A sort of housekeeping system, autophagy is your system's way to clear out dead cells and pathogens. This is good for your general health and also for your brain function.[93] You can trigger the process of autophagy not by fasting during the day, but by leaving three hours between your last meal of the day and going to bed, and not eating for 12 hours. This is far easier to achieve than starving yourself for two or more days a week. It just means you have your evening meal at 8pm, go to bed at 11pm and then have breakfast at 8am. Alternatively, some researchers suggest that you can trigger autophagy by fasting for 16 hours each day and eating within an 8 hour time slot. To achieve this you would eat only between 12pm and 8pm every day. My feeling, though, is that a 12 hour overnight (sleeping) fast is enough.

11. Understand gluten

It has become very fashionable over the last few years for people to avoid gluten which is found in rye, barley, wheat and other forms of wheat such as spelt, durum and bulgur. The question is: do you need to do this and how important is it in terms of your brain function?

Research shows that non-coeliac gluten sensitivity (see box, opposite) can upset the balance of bacteria in your gut, cause inflammation in the brain, increase cognitive dysfunction and increase a person's vulnerability to Alzheimer's.[94] So, avoiding gluten could be important in terms of preventing and treating cognitive decline. If you are going to be tested then it is important not to remove gluten before the test as this will affect your result. It is recommended that you eat gluten every day for at least six weeks before the test.

Testing for coeliac disease and non-coeliac gluten sensitivity is covered in Chapter 13.

Gluten and intolerance

There are several conditions in which gluten is an issue for the human body. The main ones are:

- **Coeliac disease.** An auto-immune response, coeliac disease is not an allergy to gluten (found in grains including wheat, barley and rye), but a disease that damages the lining of the small intestines, flattening down the villi so that the body finds it harder to absorb the nutrients from food. This can lead to weight loss, anaemia, diarrhoea, mouth ulcers and abdominal pain.

- **Non-coeliac gluten sensitivity.** If you test negatively for coeliac disease, and there is no damage to the villi in your intestines, but eating gluten triggers symptoms similar to those for coeliac disease, you may be diagnosed with non-coeliac gluten sensitivity. The scientists define non-coeliac gluten sensitivity as 'the presence of a variety of symptoms related to gluten ingestion in patients in whom coeliac disease and wheat allergy have been excluded'.[95] Research suggests that up to 10 per cent of people could suffer from non-coeliac gluten sensitivity, compared with 1 per cent for coeliac disease.[96]

- **Wheat allergy.** A wheat allergy is just that – a reaction to wheat, but not to gluten. So, a person with a wheat allergy can eat all the other gluten grains.

Chapter 7

Step 1 (b):
Sugar and your brain health

Cases of type 2 diabetes in the UK have risen by a colossal 450 per cent since 1960 and talk of Alzheimer's being type 3 diabetes – because of its link to insulin resistance (see p.35) – shows how serious this is for our cognitive health.

The problem is, I am in no doubt, to do with sugar consumption. It makes absolute sense that a problem with blood sugar must be linked to the amount of sugar that we eat. However, many experts have argued that the real problem is the amount of fat in our diets, not sugar. Their argument is that 'fat is fattening' and being overweight increases your risk of type 2 diabetes. Slowly but surely, though, opinions are changing, with diabetes experts acknowledging that while being overweight does increase your risk of type 2 diabetes, it's the weight gain from excess sugar that's the problem, not from eating fat.

To recap, type 2 diabetes occurs when your body struggles to cope with the sugar in your blood stream. Instead of being turned into fuel, the sugar builds up because insulin receptors on your cells fail to send the signals that your system needs to move sugar out of your blood and into your cells as fuel. This is called insulin resistance, which as we already know is a risk factor for Alzheimer's (see p.35).

If a low or no sugar diet can reverse type 2 diabetes or reduce your risk of it, then it may also prevent the progression of Alzheimer's. Recent research has focused on getting people with type 2 diabetes to consume no more than 25 per cent of their calories from carbohydrates, a 'hidden' source of sugar. According to Diabetes UK, over the course of six months, 70 per cent of the participants successfully lowered their blood sugar levels.

If you have a sweet tooth, the thought of giving up sugar may seem daunting. In my clinic a lot of people say they will never be able to give it up! However, you will be surprised how quickly your taste buds change and how you come to appreciate the natural sweetness of foods. Here are some ways to reduce your sugar intake.

Think before you drink

A lot of sugary calories are consumed in fizzy drinks. One European study found that just one sugar-sweetened drink a day increases your risk of type 2 diabetes by 22 per cent.[97] Interestingly, pure fruit juices – almost equally as high in sugar (albeit natural sugar) – do not seem to have the same effect, according to this study. However, artificial sweeteners – which you may assume to be the safe option – also increase your risk.

Research from France, tracking more than 66,000 women over 14 years, found that the risk of developing type 2 diabetes was higher for those who drank either artificially sweetened or sugar-sweetened drinks. However, the really interesting part was that the risk was actually highest among those drinking the artificially sweetened drinks, with 500ml a week increasing risk by 15 per cent, but 1.5 litres causing a 59 per cent higher risk. This study again showed no link between drinking 100 per cent fruit juices and the risk of diabetes.[98]

Sugar and Alzheimer's

Almost three quarters of people – a staggering 70 per cent – with type 2 diabetes are now known to develop Alzheimer's, compared with only 10 per cent of people without diabetes. In lab studies this phenomenon has been borne out, with animals bred to develop type 2 diabetes suffering a rapid deterioration in their ability to concentrate as the disease progresses. The high levels of insulin in these animals blocked a group of enzymes that would normally break down the beta-amyloid proteins responsible for the brain plaques in Alzheimer's. As it builds up, beta-amyloid forms toxic clumps (plaque) that hamper neurological function.[99]

Although high levels of insulin can have this effect, confusingly the brain also *needs* insulin for its cells to flourish and survive. Your brain has its own supply of insulin – if this supply is hampered in any way and levels of insulin in the brain fall, brain degeneration is the result. So, as with most things in Nature, we don't want too much or too little of something – it's all about homeostasis; that is, balance.

Post-mortem research on the brains of people with Alzheimer's has shown a marked reduction in insulin levels in the hippocampus, the part of the brain that the disease first affects. By contrast, the cerebellum, which Alzheimer's does not affect, did not have the same low insulin level.[100]

It's thought that changes in insulin function in the brain are the cause of beta-amyloid plaque build-up. Beta-amyloid itself is not a problem. In fact, it has a vital role to play in transporting cholesterol, protecting against oxidative stress, and aiding immune function. Problems occur only when the beta-amyloid proteins start to form clumps.

As well as helping you to regulate your blood sugar, insulin regulates neurotransmitters, brain chemicals that aid learning and memory. If you become insulin resistant, not only will your body struggle to control its blood sugar, but your neurotransmitters will be unable to function as normal, with fallout for your brain function. Studies showing the effects of insulin resistance on the brain support the importance of reducing sugar in your diet and show that just having higher levels of sugar (glucose) from eating too much sugary food is a risk factor for dementia, even if you don't have diabetes.[101]

In fact, sugar's impact on the brain goes beyond the effects of insulin. Being on the blood sugar roller coaster also increases levels of the stress hormone cortisol, and this, over time, increases inflammation in the brain, speeding up the deterioration of brain and memory function.

Spring clean your cupboards

Clear out temptation. Biscuits, chocolates and sweets are all for the local food bank. And remember that you'll find sugar in savoury foods, too – pasta sauces, soups, ketchup, breakfast cereals and many more are all culprits. If you have a sweet tooth, the hidden sugars in savoury foods will be easiest to give up first. Replace them with your own homemade salad dressings, pasta sauces, soups, granola and so on. Grit your teeth and be ruthless with those cupboard stocks.

Stop adding sugar to drinks and food

You may be doing this on autopilot, the way some people salt their food before tasting it. If you still take sugar in tea or coffee, for example, wean yourself off it half a teaspoon at a time. If you sprinkle sugar on your pancakes or cereal in the morning, try a handful of fresh berries instead. Your taste buds will adapt surprisingly quickly.

Read the labels as you shop

Every 4g of sugar per 'serving size' is 1 teaspoon of sugar. The NHS says that added sugar can comprise up to 5 per cent of your daily calorie intake – that's 30g (7 teaspoons) a day. The World Health Organisation (WHO) wants to limit added sugar (including honey) to just 6 teaspoons a day. I say to keep it as low as possible – no added sugar should be the ideal 80 per cent of the time, and then the other 20 per cent on special treats at special times won't matter.

You'll need to get sugar savvy because even something that might appear to be a healthy food, such as a fruit yogurt, can contain up to 8 teaspoons of added sugar (not including the fruit). When a food label lists its ingredients, these are in order of size, with the largest coming first. But it could be that many of these ingredients are sugar, even if the word itself doesn't feature. I've copied this label from a packet of jelly sweets. *Glucose Syrup, Sugar, Dextrose, Gelatine, Citric Acid, Caramelised Sugar Syrup, Flavourings, Fruit & Plant Concentrates (Apple, Aronia, Blackcurrant, Elderberry, Grape, Kiwi, Lemon, Mango, Nettle, Orange, Passion Fruit, Spinach), Colours (Carmine, Copper Complexes of Chlorophyll), Glazing Agents (Vegetable Oil, Beeswax, Carnauba Wax), Invert Sugar Syrup, Fruit Extract (Carob).* In this product 100g gives 63.4g of sugar – nearly 16 teaspoons. As glucose syrup, sugar and dextrose (all types of sugar) are the first three ingredients, the jellies are mainly made up of these – there's not that much else in the product. Those healthy-looking fruit extracts are minimal – a red herring to throw you off the scent of the sugar. Don't be hoodwinked!

Use your scales

It's important to know what the manufacturer's assumed serving size is compared with what you would serve yourself. For example, a 30g serving of cereal may be much smaller than you would typically eat – but if it already contains 11g sugar, how much would your own bowl contain?

Don't skip breakfast

Skipping breakfast makes you far more likely to reach for a coffee and a cake at 11am because your blood sugar will have plummeted. You may feel moody, irritable, tense and not able to concentrate. Always eat breakfast and make it a mixture of protein and carbohydrate – avoiding sugar-laden breakfast cereals at all times. For example, try a bowl of porridge (made with regular rather than quick-cook oats) sprinkled with ground nuts and seeds. The porridge oats give sustained energy and the nuts and seeds add protein to help further lower the GI. Or, have an egg (poached or scrambled) on wholemeal or rye toast with grilled tomatoes. This very low-GI breakfast provides a good amount of protein from the egg whites, omega 3 fats in the yolks, and good-quality complex, unrefined carbs from the bread – all in all a power-breakfast of energy that will sustain you until your healthy mid-morning snack (see below) and even perhaps until lunchtime. Or if you are trying to keep your carbohydrate intake low, then just have the egg with grilled tomatoes.

Eat little and often

So, you get to 3pm and you feel sluggish and tired and every part of your body is screaming to have something sweet to keep you going until teatime. Think about how you've eaten over the course of the day – did you have breakfast (see above)? Did you allow yourself a handful of nuts mid-morning? Did you eat lunch? Eating little and often is the best way to avoid blood sugar dips that lead to cravings – usually for sweet things.

Avoid extreme diets

… at least while you are trying to adapt to a no-sugar regime. This is because fasting will make it harder to avoid blood sugar dips and the cravings that come with them. Once you've cut sugar from your diet as much as you can, you'll even find that you may lose weight naturally, which will remove the need for dieting altogether.

Watch out for caffeine

This stimulant can trigger a roller coaster of stress hormones that feel a bit like sugar highs and lows. Even though it may feel like an appetite suppressant, in the end caffeine will boost your appetite and trigger sugar cravings. It's all about removing the temptation to reach for the biscuits.

Be booze aware

Alcohol has an effect on your blood sugar, so look for drinks with a lower sugar content. Spirits do not contain sugar, but their mixers usually do. White wine is more sugary than red, but on the other hand a white wine spritzer (made with sparkling mineral water) will be better for you than a full glass of red wine.

Add protein to starchy carbohydrates

If you eating starchy carbohydrates (pasta, rice, potatoes, bread), particularly if they are refined, remember that they are broken down into sugar – but protein (fish, eggs, cheese, nuts, seeds and so on) slows down the rate at which your stomach empties the food into the next part of the digestive tract and so it slows down the emptying of the carbohydrate, too. Add ground nuts and seeds to porridge for vegetable protein, or an omelette (animal protein) with brown rice.

Be kind to yourself

Live by the 80/20 rule: as long as you are eating healthily and avoiding sugar 80 per cent of the time you can have that occasional piece of cake without beating yourself up about it. This will also make it less likely you'll obsess about sugar – and fall off the wagon altogether. You're 'allowed' to have sugar 20 per cent of the time, so what's the big deal?

Be smart about alternatives

Beware 'natural' sweeteners – some may be no better for you than sugar itself. The following, though, are all worth trying:

- **Maple syrup.** This comes from the sap of maple trees and research shows it contains 34 beneficial compounds with antioxidant and anti-inflammatory properties. A number of these are polyphenols that inhibit the enzyme that converts carbohydrates into sugar and are, therefore, useful for controlling type 2 diabetes. It's also easy on the digestive system, so better than a lot of other sweeteners if you have IBS. This is not an invitation to eat as much maple syrup as you like, but it is a natural sweetener that I use (I always buy organic) in cakes and on top of crumbles. Be warned: it is expensive – so beware any cheap product or anything labelled 'maple-flavoured'. You want 100 per cent maple syrup only.

- **Barley malt syrup.** This is great for flapjacks and a good source of some minerals and vitamins. It contains almost no fructose or sucrose and is made by drying and cooking sprouted barley malt, then filtering the liquid that's left over and reducing it to a thick, dark-brown syrup. It is another good choice as a natural sweetener, especially when used in baking when the malt flavour is a bonus.

- **Brown rice syrup.** Also known as rice malt syrup, this is a health-food shop staple containing the sugars maltotriose, maltose and glucose. The best (and more expensive) types are organic and made from sprouted grains, which release enzymes that cause them to break down into these sugars. Brown rice syrup does tend to change the texture of baked foods – giving them a bit of crunch – so use it when this is a bonus, for example in a granola, crumble or flapjacks.

- **Palm sugar.** This is also known as jaggery, and is made from juice from the flowers of the palmyra palm tree that is boiled down to a syrup that is then allowed to crystallise. It's a traditional Ayurvedic ingredient and contains good amounts of B vitamins (including a plant source of B12). It also has a low glycaemic index (40) and is therefore recommended for diabetics. I like it as a natural sweetener and it can be used in cooking (a lot of Asian dishes use it) and drinks.

- **Coconut sugar.** Produced in a similar way to palm sugar (and known as coconut palm sugar), this comes from the sap of the flower buds of the coconut tree. It is rich in nutrients and is also a prebiotic, meaning that it helps to feed beneficial gut flora. Coconut sugar tastes a lot like brown sugar and you can also use it exactly the same as sugar in food and drinks. I would suggest buying organic coconut sugar.

- **Yacon syrup.** Made from the sweet root of the yacon (a member of the sunflower family, which tastes like a cross between an apple and a pear), this contains good amounts of a prebiotic called FOS (fructooligosaccharide), which helps to feed the beneficial bacteria in your gut. It's also rich in vitamins and minerals, very low GI (1) and said to be acceptable for those with diabetes. Like maple syrup, it is traditionally made without chemicals. I recommend this as a liquid sweetener, which you could use instead of honey in baking. Choose an organic variety, but bear in mind that it may not be suitable for people with IBS, owing to its high FOS content.

The following natural sugars, however, I think are better avoided:

- **Fructose Taken from fruit.** Fructose does not cause the same release of insulin as sucrose and glucose do – and that makes it look like a healthy form of sugar. However, when sold as a powder, it is totally refined and devoid of all the goodness and fibre that would have been in the fruit it came from. It also has other negative effects on your health. First, it goes straight to your liver to be metabolised in the same way as alcohol does. Fructose also triggers lipogenesis (the production of fats; that is cholesterol and triglycerides) in the liver, which can, in turn, lead to 'fatty liver' and liver damage, and also to an increased risk of heart disease. High levels of triglycerides are associated with type 2 diabetes, so it's ironic that many people switch to fructose (it has a low GI of 19) instead of sucrose in an attempt to stop insulin spikes. Research comparing the effect of fructose-sweetened drinks with glucose-sweetened drinks on obese people, found that those who had the fructose-sweetened drinks with their meals had triglyceride levels 200 per cent higher than those who drank the glucose-sweetened drinks with their food.[102]

The metabolism of fructose is twice as fast as that of glucose, so the toll on your body is greater. In addition, fructose suppresses the hormone leptin, which lets you know when you are full, limiting your control over your appetite. Watch out for the wording fructose-glucose or glucose-fructose syrup on a label in the UK as this is high fructose corn syrup which is very popular in America because it is cheaper to use than regular sugar.

High fructose corn syrup and refined fructose are known as 'unbound' or 'free' but when the fructose is contained with fruit it is bound up with the vitamins and minerals, fibre, fatty acids and other sugars within that food so it does not affect your liver in the same way.

- **Agave syrup.** The agave is a cactus native to Mexico but, when it is used to make sweetener on a commercial scale, the syrup is just as refined as fructose and made by the same process that converts corn starch into high fructose corn syrup. There may be some companies producing agave syrup in the traditional way (taking sap from the plant and boiling it for hours to obtain the syrup), but it is often difficult to tell whether any individual product is made one way or the other. This means it's safer avoided.

- **Honey.** Although it is completely natural, honey is a simple sugar, primarily made up of glucose and fructose, and this means it's absorbed into your bloodstream quickly. Some honeys may contain up to 40 per cent fructose. As a result, it is not ideal if you're trying to control your blood sugar (or lose weight), but if you do want to use it, do so sparingly.

- **Molasses.** The by-product of the process used to extract sugar from sugar cane or beet, molasses has relatively low amounts of sugar, but proportionately high quantities of vitamins and minerals. And, it's a good source of vitamin B6, potassium, magnesium and manganese. So, what's the problem? Well, being a by-product of sugar extraction, it may also have higher levels of the pesticides and other chemicals used in sugar cultivation and processing. It also has a very strong taste.

- **Xylitol.** You can buy this in a powder that looks just like sugar. It's low in calories because it occurs naturally in plants, and it doesn't need insulin to be metabolised in the body, making it very useful for diabetics. However, the extensive processing involved in making it (a process of hydrogenation of a sugar called xylose derived from the fibre of plants such as sugar cane, corn cobs and birch) is far from natural, which – for me – makes it an alternative to avoid.

- **Sorbitol.** Often used in foods designed for diabetics because it requires little or no insulin for its metabolism, sorbitol is usually made from corn syrup, but is found naturally in stone fruits such as prunes, plums and dates. It is another highly processed product and, like xylitol, the processing includes hydrogenation – which we know is unhealthy when applied to fats. Both sorbitol and xylitol can cause diarrhoea and worsen IBS for some people.

- **Stevia.** Made from the leaves of the stevia plant, this product is amazingly sweet – in fact up to 300 times sweeter than refined white sugar. Although this sounds like a good solution, many products in supermarkets claiming to be stevia also contain dextrose and flavourings. This makes it a risky choice but, if you do buy it, check labels carefully to make sure you find a product that really is 100 per cent stevia. It also acts a bit like an artificial sweetener, priming your body to expect a corresponding amount of calories for its sweetness – although it is supposed to have no calories itself. It can leave a bitter aftertaste for some people.

- **Evaporated cane juice (ECJ).** A partially purified sugar – so not quite as refined as normal white sugar – ECJ nonetheless has the same effects as refined sugar on your body. In essence, it is just another form of processed sugar, so to be avoided.

- **Artificial sweeteners.** When you see a fizzy drink labelled 'sugar free' it will often contain an artificial sweetener with no calories. No calories = no weight gain, you may think. But, in a cruel twist of fate, these artificial sweeteners send a message to your brain that you have just eaten something sweet, and your brain then tells your body to expect the calories that should have come with it. The problem with this is that you then crave sweet foods and are likely to eat them! In one study, rats given artificial sweeteners gained more weight than rats given the same number of calories in sugar.[103] Research has also shown that people who drink two or more diet drinks a day have waist circumference increases 500 per cent greater than those who don't.[104] This is a risk factor for type 2 diabetes, and, in turn, Alzheimer's. My advice is to avoid artificial sweeteners, such as aspartame, sucralose and saccharin, at all costs.

If you would like some delicious sugar-free recipes then see my book *Natural Alternatives to Sugar*, available from Amazon.

Chapter 8

Step 2: Nutritional supplements

It goes without saying that what you eat is the foundation of your health – your nutrition starts with your food. But there are also certain crucial nutrients that are really important for Alzheimer's and dementia and have been studied in the medical literature for their benefits on brain function. And, although you may think (and may indeed have been told) that you could obtain all these nutrients from diet alone, I have to say that, having now been in the nutritional field for over 30 years – and despite having once been one of those who believed food alone could provide all we need – I am now convinced that most of us will also need the extra help that nutritional supplements can provide.

Food does not always contain the nutrients it should and I think there are two main reasons why. First, owing to over-farming and the use of pesticides, UK soils are now significantly nutrient depleted. For example, some sources claim that we may have up to half the selenium levels in our soil that we should have. And, second, food loses nutrients from the moment it is picked – so if we buy foods that have travelled long distances to get to us, they arrive significantly nutritionally bereft. Fruit and vegetables contain, on average, 20 per cent fewer minerals (including magnesium, calcium, iron and zinc) than they did in the 1930s. Iron levels in meat are down by 47 per cent and in milk by more than 60 per cent. Calcium levels in cheese are down by 15 per cent; in Parmesan by 70 per cent.[105]

Also people nowadays can have malnutrition not because they don't have enough food but ironically because they have too much of the wrong kind. People can be overfed and undernourished because the food can just be empty calories with no nutritional value. They can even be overweight but still malnourished.

So, what are the key nutritional supplements you need to help prevent Alzheimer's and dementia?

Omega 3 essential fats

Your brain is 70 per cent fat and it incorporates whatever fats you eat into its cell membranes, aiming to keep the cells flexible and properly functioning. However, as we learned on page 79, not all fats have this effect. Trans fats, for example, stiffen up your brain cells, impeding their function.

Omega 3 fats, on the other hand, are the good guys. They comprise EPA (eicosapentaenoic acid) and DHA (docosahexaenoic acid), the latter accounting for 97 per cent of the omega 3 fats found in your brain and so the most important for helping to slow down the progression of Alzheimer's and dementia. DHA also accounts for up to 93 per cent of the omega 3 found in your retina. Research has shown that DHA has the most protective effective against Alzheimer's.[106]

The diagram[107] below shows how powerful DHA is in its neuroprotective effects. It can prevent amyloid plaque formation[108] and aggregation, improve cerebral blood flow and reduce inflammation, making it important in the fight against not only Alzheimer's but also vascular dementia.

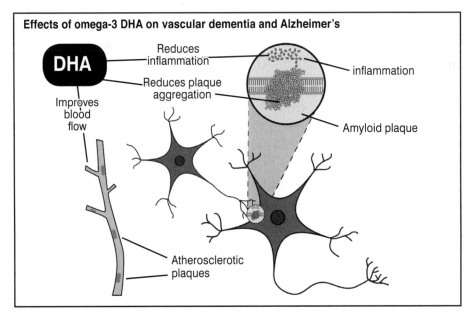

Effects of omega-3 DHA on vascular dementia and Alzheimer's

An interesting study looked at blood levels of omega 3 and MRI scans of more than 1,000 postmenopausal women over the course of eight years. They found that the hippocampus, the part of the brain that is so important for cognitive function and that shrinks with Alzheimer's, was smallest in those women who had the lowest omega 3 (EPA plus DHA) levels.[109] The higher levels of omega 3 correlated with both large brain and large hippocampal volume to the extent that the researchers have asked whether maintaining higher levels of EPA and DHA would slow the rate of shrinkage of the hippocampus over time.

Omega 3 fats are important for preventing vascular dementia because they not only help with good blood flow, as in the diagram, but they can also help to prevent abnormal blood clotting and they help lower blood pressure.[110]

For your general health the Harvard School of Public Health has stated that diets deficient in omega 3 cause up to 96,000 preventable deaths a year in the USA.[111] The researchers estimated the number of deaths resulting from 12 preventable causes and omega 3 deficiency ranked as the sixth highest killer of Americans.

There are two important things to know about omega 3.

The first is that omega 3 fats are known as 'essential' and that means your body cannot produce them, so you have to take them in either from your food or in supplement form. And, second, that we are getting proportionately too much omega 6 (see p.75).

There has been an 80 per cent decrease in the consumption of omega 3 fatty acids[112] over the last century. Deficiency symptoms can appear as dryness, such as dry and lifeless hair, painful joints, arthritis, cracked skin on heels or fingertips, dry skin and arthritis. (When you see your skin and hair improve, you can be reassured that the same processes are happening in your brain as the essential fatty acids lubricate that, too.)

That omega 3 fat deficiency has sky-rocketed is no surprise to me. The notion that 'fat is bad', particularly among women, is one that I see frequently in my clinic.

As the diagram opposite shows, if you have too much omega 6 in your system, you may be producing substances that have a pro-inflammatory effect on your body, and can also increase abnormal blood clotting. Inflammation can appear anywhere in your body, not only in your brain. Any pain, soreness, or redness anywhere – such as in your joints (as in arthritis), bowels (as in an inflammatory bowel disorder, such as ulcerative colitis and Crohn's disease) or skin (such as eczema and psoriasis) is the result of inflammation. It's easy to feel and recognise these forms of inflammation, but that's not so when the inflammation occurs in your brain. Finally, an increase in the omega 6 to omega 3 ratio can increase your risk of obesity,[113] which in turn can increases your risk of type 2 diabetes and Alzheimer's.

Where does the excess omega 6 come from?

The obvious source of omega 6 in the modern diet is processed food containing vegetable oils. However, that's not the only way we might be increasing our intake of this essential fat. Many of the women I see in my clinic have been taking evening primrose oil supplements for years, raising their levels of omega 6 and increasing the ratio of omega 6 to omega 3. Others are taking combinations such as omega 3, 6 and 9 in supplement form, because they have heard that we need a good balance of all the omega fatty acids. (This is true, but you have to take into account what your own levels may be in the first place as it is no good adding in more omega 6 if you have already got enough or, in fact, too much in your body.) Omega 9 is found in olive oil and is not classed as an essential fat because you can manufacture this in your body, unlike omega 3 and omega 6, so there is usually no need to supplement with it.

Modern farming methods also contribute to the imbalance. Many animals are fed corn (grain), which is a source of omega 6, altering the balance of fats that metabolise from the food of these animals. This means that meat from corn fed animals have higher levels of omega 6 and less omega 3 than those that are grass fed.[114]

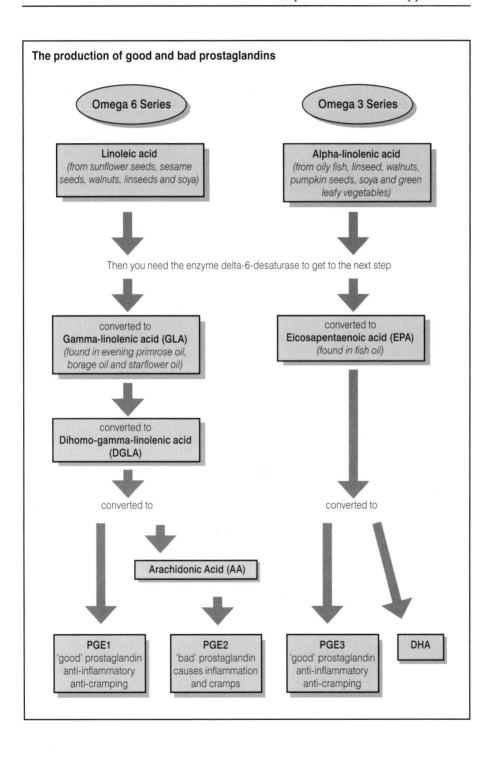

The production of good and bad prostaglandins

Omega 6 Series

Omega 3 Series

Linoleic acid
(from sunflower seeds, sesame seeds, walnuts, linseeds and soya)

Alpha-linolenic acid
(from oily fish, linseed, walnuts, pumpkin seeds, soya and green leafy vegetables)

Then you need the enzyme delta-6-desaturase to get to the next step

converted to
Gamma-linolenic acid (GLA)
(found in evening primrose oil, borage oil and starflower oil)

converted to
Eicosapentaenoic acid (EPA)
(found in fish oil)

converted to
Dihomo-gamma-linolenic acid (DGLA)

converted to

converted to

Arachidonic Acid (AA)

PGE1
'good' prostaglandin
anti-inflammatory
anti-cramping

PGE2
'bad' prostaglandin
causes inflammation
and cramps

PGE3
'good' prostaglandin
anti-inflammatory
anti-cramping

DHA

Boosting omega 3 through supplements

First and foremost, I recommend that everyone has a simple finger prick test to establish their ratio and levels of omega 3 to omega 6 fatty acids, so that you know how much omega 3 you need to boost (and omega 6 to reduce). This is particularly important if you are vegetarian or vegan (see p.76).

What to choose: omega 3 fish oils

Bear in mind when you are reading the label of an omega 3 supplement: it is not the amount of omega 3 it contains that matters, but the amount of EPA and DHA. Unless you are vegetarian, take an omega 3 fish oil supplement containing 770mg EPA and 510mg DHA (the one I use in my clinic is NHP's Omega 3 Support; see www.naturalhealthpractice.com. I don't use any cod liver oil supplements in my clinic, because the oil extracted from the liver of the fish (rather than the body) can contain high quantities of heavy metals or toxins. In 2006, in the UK two companies had to remove their cod liver oil capsules from the shelves because they contained toxic dioxins (a carcinogen) at a level above the legal limit. When you're choosing an omega 3 supplement, therefore, check that the oils come from the body of the fish.

And try and make sure that the supplement you choose comes from wild, rather than farmed, fish and small fish, such as anchovies and sardines. Large fish, such as tuna, can contain high levels of mercury. You can get some vegetarian EPA and DHA supplements, but they usually don't contain high enough levels.

Types of omega 3 fish oil

I mentioned above about checking the amount of EPA and DHA within the supplement you are choosing; but there is also something else that you need to check and that is the form of the omega 3 oil.

It's not just the amount of EPA and DHA within the supplement you need to check when you choose an omega 3 supplement.

You need to check the form of the omega 3 oil and they are not all the same and the difference is really important to your health.

Omega 3 oils have three main forms. They are:

- Phospholipids
- Ethyl esters
- Triglycerides

Below, I look at omega 3 supplements taken from krill, which comes in the phospholipid form. I don't advise taking this kind of omega 3 supplement; read on to see why. Then, ethyl ester forms of omega 3 fish oil are synthetic and based in alcohol. They are the cheapest form of fish oil to produce, but they are also the least bio-available. As your body usually ingests fats in the triglyceride form it means that if you take in an oil in the ethyl ester form your body has to rebuild this fat back into a triglyceride. Research has shown that the triglyceride fish oils are better absorbed than the ethyl ester forms. Ethyl esters are also less stable than triglyceride fish oils and so can oxidise, creating free radicals in your body.

This means, then, that the triglyceride is the most natural form – it is the form in which you would absorb omega 3 oils from eating the fish. In fact, more than 98 per cent of all fats are triglycerides. Overall, when you're choosing an omega 3 fish oil supplement, choose the one with triglyceride on its label.

Krill oil supplements

I must mention krill oil because there has been such media hype about it. As I've said, when you eat fish, you absorb the omega 3 fat in the triglyceride form. Those who advocate krill oil supplementation claim that it is superior to fish oil because it comes in the phospholipid form, which manufacturers say the body finds easier to absorb.

A study in 2013 suggested that krill oil could be more effective than fish oil at improving omega 3 levels and reducing the omega 6 to omega 3 ratio.[115] Then, in 2014, researchers said that the study was flawed, because the scientists did not use a typical fish oil (which is high in omega 3), but an oil high in omega 6 fatty acids, skewing the results.

Other scientists made this comment: 'Due to the fatty acid profile being non-representative of typically commercially marketed fish oil, the conclusions presented by Rasmprasath et al are not justified and [are] misleading. Considerable care is needed in ensuring that such comparative trials do not use inappropriate ingredients.'[116]

The EPA and DHA in krill oil supplements is very low. For about 2,000mg krill you get around 240mg EPA and 110mg DHA. The same amount of fish oil supplement gives about 770mg EPA and 510mg DHA. Still further controversy arrived in 2014 when research re-examined the studies which have looked at the bioavailability of krill oil – that is how easily krill oil is absorbed into your body. They point out that it has proven difficult to compare the bioavailability of krill oil versus fish oil because of the lower concentrations of both EPA and DHA in krill oil compared to fish oil. They also point to other factors that have made it difficult to compare the two and conclude 'that there is at present no evidence for greater bioavailability of krill oil versus fish oil'.[117]

It wasn't until the scientists designed a study comparing krill to fish oil using the same amount of EPA and DHA that we could see that as long as you compared like with like, then you got similar rises in blood levels of EPA and DHA.[118] But you would need to take at least three times as much of the krill oil to match the levels of EPA and DHA in fish oil.

One well known supplement company who sells krill oil has now 'fortified' (their words) their krill oil supplement with fish oil on their 'nutritionists' advice'. To me, it just makes more sense to take fish oil in the first place.

Finally, my last concern about krill oil is an ecological one. Krill is not a fish but a crustacean and it is the bottom of the food chain for many animals, including whales, fish, seals and seabirds. It seems that the whole Antarctic ecosystem revolves around it. Some health food stores have taken krill oil off the shelves because of the decline in certain sea animals, whales, penguins and seals where the krill is harvested.

B vitamins

The B vitamins, in particular vitamins B6 and B12 and folic acid, help to control an amino acid, called homocysteine that occurs naturally in your body, but has a toxic effect when the level is too high. Although your body should detoxify homocysteine, if that does not happen then this can lead to high circulating levels, which some research suggests 'is a strong, independent risk factor for the development of dementia and Alzheimer's'. In the research study, if the level of homocysteine was found to be greater than 14 mmol/L from a blood test, it doubled the risk of the person developing Alzheimer's.[119]

You need good levels of the B vitamins to detoxify this amino acid. Research has shown that people taking 20mg of vitamin B6, 500mcg of vitamin B12, and 800mcg of folic acid had 90 per cent less brain shrinkage compared to those using a placebo.[120]

The protection against brain atrophy occurred in the brain areas that Alzheimer's usually destroys. The researchers state that 'B vitamin treatment reduces, by as much as seven fold, the cerebral atrophy in those grey matter regions specifically vulnerable to the Alzheimer's disease process, including the medial temporal lobe' and 'our results show that B vitamin supplementation can slow the atrophy of specific brain regions that are a key component of the Alzheimer's disease process and that are associated with cognitive decline'.

Dr Gwenaëlle Douaud, an imaging and neuroscience expert and leader of the study, says: 'We know some people with mild cognitive impairment will go on to develop Alzheimer's and the best marker of raised risk at the moment is the amount of shrinkage in an area called the medial temporal lobe. This is right in the middle of the Alzheimer's footprint – the area B vitamins protect.'

Previous research in 2010 also showed that B vitamins slowed the rate of accelerated brain shrinkage in mild cognitive impairment.[121] Interestingly, the greatest benefit was seen in those who started with the highest homocysteine level, greater than 13 mmol/L. The ones given the B vitamins with a high homocysteine level had a 53 per cent lower rate of brain atrophy than those who also had high homocysteine, but were given a placebo. Those who had the greatest rate of atrophy had the lowest final cognitive test scores.

The importance of having good levels of omega 3 is now even greater when we look at the benefits of the B vitamins, because we now know that the beneficial effects of the B vitamin supplements is found only in those people who also have good levels of omega 3 fatty acids. The rate of brain shrinkage was reduced by 73 per cent in those people who were given B vitamins but who started with a high omega 3 and a raised homocysteine.[122] They are also thinking that the beneficial effects of increased omega 3 on brain atrophy may also depend on the person having good levels of B vitamins. That is, that the benefits are mutual.

More research has shown that when omega 3 fatty acid concentrations are low, particularly when there are low levels of DHA, vitamin B supplementation has no effect on cognitive decline, but when omega 3 levels are in the upper normal range, B vitamins interact to slow cognitive decline.[123]

This is so important, because it confirms that nutrients work together to provide optimal health – which means we need to make sure we're not deficient in any nutrient, not just one or two.

Folic acid versus folate

This is the hot topic of the moment: should you take a supplement containing folic acid or should it be in the form of folate? When you eat food, you get folic acid in the form of folate – but most of the supplements provide it in the folic acid form. Indeed, the research on Alzheimer's using B vitamins talks about folic acid rather than folate.

Everybody knows that folic acid is important for a healthy pregnancy and newborn – because it helps prevent neural tube defects, such as spina bifida, in the baby. And, as we have seen, it is important together with vitamins B6 and vitamin B12 to lower circulating levels of homocysteine.

When you take folic acid in supplement form, your body converts it to l-methylfolate. However, some people have a genetic variation that makes it difficult for them to make the conversion.

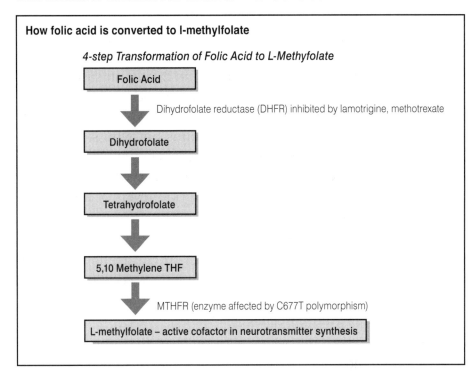

How folic acid is converted to l-methylfolate

4-step Transformation of Folic Acid to L-Methyfolate

Folic Acid

↓ Dihydrofolate reductase (DHFR) inhibited by lamotrigine, methotrexate

Dihydrofolate

↓

Tetrahydrofolate

↓

5,10 Methylene THF

↓ MTHFR (enzyme affected by C677T polymorphism)

L-methylfolate – active cofactor in neurotransmitter synthesis

As you can see in the diagram, the enzyme needed to make the last step of the conversion to methylfolate, the active folate, is controlled by an enzyme called MTHFR (methylenetetrahydrofolate reductase). A mutation in the MTHFR gene could affect how much folate you have.

Natural folate in foods is quite unstable and sensitive to oxidation and light so is not used in supplements in that form. In your body folate cannot be stored and is water soluble and is constantly being lost so needs to be replaced.

Supplements have tended to use folate in the form of folic acid as it is stable. In your body folic acid is converted to methylfolate and this is dependent on the enzyme MTHFR.

Therefore methylfolate is more bioavailable than folic acid. Until fairly recently methylfolate was not available in the UK for use in food supplements but only in medicines.

The research shows that it is necessary to use methylfolate supplements only if you have the MTHFR variant that hampers the conversion from folic acid to folate. My understanding is that the MTHFR variant affects around 12 per cent of Caucasians worldwide, although the statistics vary wildly from country to country. In Italy, for example, the variant is present in around 20 per cent of the population, while in Mexico it is found in 36 per cent.[124] You can be tested for the most common MTHFR variant C677T to see if you have it. A recent review of the scientific research suggests that the MTHFR C677T variant is associated with an increased risk of Alzheimer's.[125] (There are more than fifty MTHFR variants, including A1298C, but there is less research available on the others.) Your results will show one of three things:

- CC: Wild type – you have normal MTHFR enzyme activity and can convert folic acid to folate easily.

- CT: You have one copy of the gene variant, so you have lower conversion activity.

- TT: You have two copies of the gene variant, so your enzyme activity is very low.

You could also have a simple home finger-prick test to establish your homocysteine levels (see p.161). If they are normal, then you are unlikely to have a problem with an MTHFR variant.

Can we have too much folic acid?

Although folic acid is an important nutrient, there are concerns that having too much could increase your risk of cancer. Even though there have been concerns about fortifying flour with folic acid in the UK, the USA has been doing so since 1998 and research has shown that this has not had a negative impact on cancer risk.[126] (Although it may mask a vitamin-B12 deficiency.)

I think it is better if you can take supplements containing methylfolate rather than folic acid. If you can't then I do think it is worthwhile checking your homocysteine levels. If they come out too high, it's worth supplementing extra B vitamins for three months and then having another test. If your homocysteine levels are still high, it would be good to see what MTHFR variant you have.

What to choose: B vitamins

As well as establishing whether it's better to take folic acid or folate, choose a B vitamin supplement that provides vitamin B6 as pyridoxal-5-phosphate (P-5-P). This is the active form of B6. If you choose a B6 supplement in the form of pyridoxine (which is a much cheaper version), your body has to convert it into P-5-P in order to get the benefit. If you are run down, tired or stressed, your body may not be able to make the conversion from pyridoxine to P-5-P, so you don't get the benefit of having taken the supplement.

L-arginine

An essential amino acid, l-arginine produces nitric oxide, an important neurotransmitter that is thought to be one of the chemical messengers involved in learning and memory.[127] Research has suggested that 'l-arginine may play a prominent role in the treatment of age-related degenerative disease such as Alzheimer's.'[128] We know that l-arginine, which produces nitric oxide, can help to improve cognitive function in people with dementia.[129]

Nitric oxide expands your blood vessels, improves blood flow and decreases abnormal blood clotting, all important actions to protect you against heart disease, but also to protect you against vascular dementia.

Acetyl-l-carnitine

An amino acid that increases the activity of the brain receptors that normally deteriorate with age, according to research, acetyl-l-carnitine 'appears to have neuroprotective properties and it has recently been shown to reduce attention deficits in patients with Alzheimer's disease'.[130] We know that people with Alzheimer's have significantly lower levels of acetyl-l-carnitine compared to people without this disease.[131]

Acetyl-l-carnitine works with co-enzyme Q10 and alpha lipoic acid (see below) to maintain the function of the mitochondria – the cellular power houses that provide the energy for your cells to function and survive.

People with Alzheimer's have been found to have a shortage of the neurotransmitter acetylcholine in the brain and drugs that mimic acetylcholine are often used as a treatment for Alzheimer's, but only 30–40 per cent of Alzheimer's patients actually respond to the treatment. So researchers used a combination treatment with the drug and acetyl-l-carnitine and found that the usual response rate with the acetylcholinesterase inhibitor was 38 per cent but this increased to 50 per cent with the addition of acetyl-l-carnitine. In other words, a nutrient is making the drug treatment more effective.[132]

Alpha lipoic acid

A powerful antioxidant that is both water and fat soluble and so readily absorbed by your body (including your brain), alpha lipoid acid plays a major role in controlling blood sugar because it burns glucose to make energy. Furthermore, alpha lipoic acid can help to increase your body's production of acetylcholine, which we know is low in those with Alzheimer's;[133] and help prevent high blood pressure, which is important for those who are susceptible to vascular dementia.[134]

Phosphatidyl choline

Your body uses phosphatidyl choline to make the brain chemical acetylcholine, which occurs in low levels in people with Alzheimer's. Research on animals with dementia has shown that giving phosphatidyl choline increases the concentration of acetylcholine in the brain and improves memory[135] and that phosphatidylcholine can protect neurons from the toxic effects of beta-amyloid.[136]

As one study pointed out 'both DHA and phosphatidylcholine have been shown to halt the pathogenesis of Alzheimer disease and vascular dementia'.[137] Then, the researchers wondered what would happen if the two were combined. They found that the combination of the two nutrients significantly improved the learning and memory abilities of the rats.

Phosphatidylserine

An important part of all your cells, but particularly the cell membrane, phosphatidylserine has been shown to improve vocabulary and picture-matching scores in Alzheimer's patients. In rats, phosphatidylserine improved memory and reduced levels of cholinesterase.[138] Research has shown that phosphatidylserine and omega 3 together can improve memory and cognitive performance in all people – not only those who have a diagnosis of Alzheimer's or dementia.[139]

Combining supplements

Taking a programme of supplements that gives you specific combinations of nutrients is often more effective than taking a few individual nutrients, because nutrients work not only individually, but synergistically with each other. So a combined supplement programme is greater than the sum of its parts. When researchers used a combination of alphalipoic acid, acetyl-l-carnitine, DHA and phosphatidylserine, they found that not only did it reduce free radicals by 57 per cent, but it also prevented marked cognitive decline. 'These findings add to the growing body of research indicating that key dietary supplementation may delay the progression of age-related cognitive decline.'[140]

I use a supplement in my clinic called Advanced Brain and Memory Support. This contains the level of B vitamins used in the research on p.107, folic acid in the active methylfolate form, vitamin D3, phosphatidylserine, phosphatidyl choline, acetyl-l-carnitine, alpha lipoic acid, l-arginine, tyrosine, zinc, co-enzyme Q10, vitamin A, vitamin E and selenium.   (See NHP's Advanced Brain and Memory Support www.naturalhealthpractice.com).

Zinc

An important immune-boosting antioxidant, zinc is a crucial mineral for brain health if an immune-system malfunction contributes to the build-up of beta-amyloid plaques. Research shows that people with Alzheimer's are often zinc deficient compared with age-matched people without the disease.[141] And there is an opposite relationship between zinc and copper (the latter of which can come from tapwater, among other sources): the higher the levels of copper in the body, the lower the levels of zinc.

Zinc supplementation has been shown to protect against cognitive loss and lower copper levels and the 'efficacy may come from restoring normal zinc levels, or from lowering serum free copper, or from both'.[142]

Vitamin D

We have known for many years that vitamin D is important for bone health and in the prevention of osteoporosis. However, it is only in recent years that we have realised how important this nutrient is for general health and, particularly, for brain health. Here are just some of the main benefits of vitamin D:

- It in plays a major role in breast and bowel cancer prevention.

- It is important for your immune function, particularly when you need to fight off colds and flu.

- It helps protect your body against conditions as diverse as type 2 diabetes, heart disease, joint pains and arthritis, dementia, infertility, autism and allergies.

- It reduces the risk of SAD (Seasonal Affective Disorder).

Vitamin D deficiencies have also been implicated in autoimmune diseases, such as rheumatoid arthritis, lupus and inflammatory bowel disease.

We get most of our vitamin D quota from sunlight, because natural food sources are few. Those most at risk of vitamin D deficiency are those who do not go out much in the daytime, those who do not expose their skin to the sunlight, and women who constantly wear make-up or cosmetics with in-built sun protection factors. The tone of your skin affects vitamin D production, so the darker your skin the less your body produces vitamin D. Covering up large areas of skin for religious reasons also reduces vitamin D production. It is estimated that we need about 30 minutes exposure to the sun every day to produce enough vitamin D to keep us healthy – but it has to be the right kind of sun.

Your body produces the best levels of vitamin D when you are exposed to sunlight within a specific UVB spectrum. In certain parts of the UK, such as northern England, Northern Ireland and Scotland, the sunlight is in the wrong spectrum for most of the year.

Vitamin D in food

Food sources of vitamin D are relatively few. It is found in oily fish and eggs (a 100g of grilled salmon contains 284ius of vitamin D and a 100g of tinned pilchards contains 560ius, the yolk of one egg contains about 20ius). Other sources include fortified foods such as margarines and breakfast cereals.

Vitamin D deficiency has become such an issue in the UK (we now have rickets, which we thought we'd eliminated over 40 years ago) that the advice from the Scientific Advisory Committee on Nutrition recommends that adults and children take vitamin D in supplement form (400ius,10mcg) every day, especially over the winter.

If you are moderately deficient in vitamin D, you have a 53 per cent increased risk of dementia, and your risk increases by 125 per cent if you are severely deficient. With Alzheimer's, one study found that those who were moderately deficient had a 69 per cent increased risk, and the risk increased to 122 per cent in those who were severely deficient.[143] This research showed evidence that there seems to be a threshold level in the blood below which the risk of developing dementia and Alzheimer's increases. Levels above 50 nmol/L are the most strongly associated with good brain health. I think a level between 80 and 100 nmol/L gives the best overall effect on general health and this is level I get my patients to aim for in my clinic.

Symptoms of vitamin D deficiency

The symptoms of a vitamin D deficiency are very subtle (bone pain, muscle weakness) and you may not suspect that lack of vitamin D is the issue. The only way to know for sure is to have a blood test (a home finger-prick test is available; see p.172), supplement if needed and then retest about three months later to make sure your level is within the optimal range.

A question a lot of people ask me when I give talks, is how much vitamin D should they take? The answer, of course, is that it depends on the level of your deficiency. For this reason, I now recommend that everyone gets their vitamin D level checked given this nutrient's far-reaching health benefits and then to supplement to get the level back to normal. We have had instances in the clinic where the lab has phoned to say there was no vitamin D detected at all.

There is, though, such a thing as too much vitamin D. A vitamin D level that is too low (less than 10 nmol/L) increases the risk of all-cause mortality (dying of any cause) – but the same is true if your vitamin D level is too high (more than 140 nmol/L).[144] Similarly, a level of vitamin D that is too low or too high increases an allergic response, such as the response you'd have during a peanut or shellfish allergy.[145]

Vitamin D balances your immune function (if you have an autoimmune problem it's especially important to have your vitamin D levels tested), helps control inflammation, has antioxidant properties and helps to control beta-amyloid plaque build-up.[146] All these benefits are important for your brain health, so getting your levels just right is crucial if you are to benefit from them.

What to choose: vitamin D

Choose vitamin D in the form of D3, also called cholecalciferol. There is a cheaper form, called D2 (ergocalciferol), but research suggests that vitamin D3 is 87 per cent more effective at raising and maintaining your vitamin D levels than vitamin D2.[147] Researchers have said that 'the assumption that vitamins D2 and D3 have equal nutritional value is probably wrong and should be reconsidered'. Most people (especially older people) do not convert vitamin D2 to the active form that their bodies can use efficiently.

Antioxidants

In Chapter 6 we looked at how important it is to eat a wide range of fruit and vegetables because the antioxidants they supply help control free radical damage in your body and brain. You can also get antioxidants in supplement form.

Combined antioxidant supplements

Most antioxidant supplements include the vitamins A, C and E and the minerals zinc and selenium. Some combinations may include other antioxidants, such as co-enzyme Q10 and alpha lipoic acid. You can make these in your body, although levels fall as you get older.

We know that combinations of vitamins C and E in supplement form are associated with a reduced risk of Alzheimer's.[148] However, of particular interest to me, is the finding that the reduction in risk does not exist if the vitamins are taken separately – the benefits in terms of Alzheimer's risk appears to occur only when the vitamin supplements are taken together, reinforcing the notion that nutrients work together to their best effects.

Vitamin C

Unlike most animals (but like apes and guinea pigs), we can't manufacture vitamin C in our bodies – it has to come from our diet or from supplements. Vitamin C levels can be lower in people with Alzheimer's. Research on mice supports the notion that there is a link between vitamin C and dementia because it has shown that vitamin C supplementation can reduce beta-amyloid plaque build-up.[149] Furthermore, some research suggests that the breaking down of the blood–brain barrier is a factor in the progression of the disease and we know that vitamin C helps with keeping the integrity of the barrier between your blood and brain.

Vitamin C and stress

Stress depletes our stores of vitamin C. Animals that can manufacture their own vitamin C, in the liver and kidneys, do so when they are stressed, replenishing stocks to restore health. Because the human body can't make its own vitamin C, you need to make sure that, during times of anxiety, you supplement your own stocks not only with increased intake of vitamin C rich foods, but also with a supplement.

Vitamin C is important for glucose metabolism, which is essential for keeping your blood-sugar levels stable. Research has shown that 1000mg of vitamin C a day for just six weeks can help decrease blood glucose (sugar), insulin, HbAlc and LDL ('bad') cholesterol levels in people with type 2 diabetes. Taking 500mg a day did not make any difference.[150]

Vitamin C can also be helpful if you need to lose weight. If you have good levels of vitamin C you will burn 30 per cent more fat when you're doing moderate exercise than someone with low levels of the vitamin. It is thought that when vitamin C levels are low, the body slows down fat burning as a safety measure.

I recommend taking 500mg vitamin C twice a day (because this vitamin is water soluble, it is better taken in two amounts, as your body can't store the excess of a single amount). Choose an alkaline form, such as magnesium ascorbate, which is gentler on your digestive system than ascorbic acid (see NHP's Vitamin C Support www.naturalhealthpractice.com).

Resveratrol

Found in the skin of red grapes, resveratrol is an antioxidant nutrient currently under investigation for its benefits in relation to slowing the onset of Alzheimer's.[151] Greater amounts of resveratrol are present in red wine and red grape juice than in the white versions, because the nutrient-rich grape skin is left intact to make red wine and juice. Peanuts and berries are also good sources.

What to choose: antioxidants

Choose an antioxidant supplement that contains vitamin E in the form of d-alpha-tocopherol. This is the natural version of vitamin E; dl-alpha-tocopherol is the synthetic version and your body doesn't absorb it as easily. Furthermore, choose vitamin C ascorbate (magnesium ascorbate). This is the alkaline rather than the acidic form (ascorbic acid) and is much gentler on your digestive system.

Serrapeptase

Research into the efficacy of serrapeptase in relation to Alzheimer's is scarce at the moment, but the first signs are positive – which is why it warrants a place in this book.[152]

An enzyme found in the digestive system of silkworms, serrapeptase destroys protein (proteolytic) to dissolve the silkworm's cocoon. Scientists hypothesise that, in humans, serrapeptase can break down non-living tissue such as scar tissue and blood clots, and that it has anti-inflammatory effects.

Dementia is characterised by the build-up of protein (beta-amyloid) plaques in the brain. Scientists hope that serrapeptase can work on these proteins as it does on those of the cocoon. Although we know that addressing the underlying cause of the beta-amyloid build-up is the most important way in which to try to slow the progression of cognitive decline, taking supplements of serrapeptase can potentially help to break down plaques that are already there. While we need more research, I see no reason why taking supplements of this enzyme couldn't help, alongside improved diet and lifestyle, and better-researched supplementation. Be careful, though, if you are taking any medication that slows down blood clotting, such as warfarin (an anti-coagulant), as it is thought that serrapeptase might also have an anti-coagulant effect, putting you at risk of bleeding or bruising.

Calcium

The situation with regard to calcium is complex. Research has suggested that women who've had a stroke and take calcium supplements for five years have an increased risk of vascular dementia.[153] The risk was there only in women who'd had a stroke or who had damage to their blood vessels showing poor blood flow in the brain. However, this was a small study: the researchers point out that the risk was there only in six women out of 15 who had had a stroke and were taking calcium supplements. With those who'd had other damage to the brain, not a stroke, 50 out of 316 women taking calcium supplements had an increased risk of dementia.

Because of the small numbers, we'd need the study repeated to be more confident in the findings.

If you intend to take calcium supplements, make sure your vitamin D levels are at their optimum, as your body needs vitamin D to absorb and use calcium efficiently. Also, unless you are prescribed calcium in the form of calcium carbonate, avoid this form of the mineral. Calcium carbonate is chalk – an inorganic form that is not like the calcium you eat in your food. Instead, take the organic form calcium citrate, which is how calcium is found in food and is, therefore, more easily absorbed into the body.

One study suggests that calcium supplements 'are associated with a higher risk of myocardial infarction and cardiovascular events'[154] and others are concerned that it speeds the process of calcification of the blood vessel, impeding blood flow around the body and in the brain. However, these hypotheses are inconclusive because the type of calcium and the form in which it was supplemented was not clear.

Probiotics

Over the last few years, research into probiotics and how these beneficial bacteria can affect our health has exploded – proving that probiotics have a far more significant effect on our whole body than only the positive effects on your gut health. Your brain and gut are very much connected and good bacteria have direct effects on your memory, mood and cognition.[155] Scientists talk about the brain–gut axis; and they even call the gut the 'second brain', because it is filled with the same neurotransmitters as your brain.

Your digestive system contains billions of bacteria (good and bad), weighing in at around 1kg (about 2lbs). You need good levels of beneficial bacteria (probiotics) to help to keep control of the pathogenic bacteria, parasites and yeasts. There is a delicate bacterial balance to be had and keeping that balance is extremely important for your overall good health. Probiotics manufacture the B vitamins and vitamin K and improve digestive function. They are also important for immunity, as 70 per cent of the immune system is in your gut, and we know they can alleviate[156] and prevent allergic diseases, such as hay fever, food intolerances and eczema. Beneficial bacteria improve detoxification (including heavy metals) which is crucial for brain health and, through their role improving digestion, prevent food sitting in the gut producing toxins. Both probiotics and prebiotics (they promote the growth of the probiotics) have anti-inflammatory effects,[157] which we know is important in the treatment of both vascular dementia and Alzheimer's. Overall, 'probiotic bacteria represent the most promising intervention for primary prevention'.[158]

Unfortunately, the natural levels of probiotics fall as we get older. In addition, they are reduced in number, or even wiped out totally, if we use antibiotics or HRT. The contraceptive pill and stress also deplete them.

Gut bacteria and weight control

Your gut flora can help control whether you gain weight[159] and can influence your risk of becoming insulin resistant or developing type 2 diabetes.[160] We know that being overweight is linked to a higher risk of Alzheimer's and that insulin resistance affects whether your brain gets the energy it needs from your food in order to function efficiently.

Research has indicated that changing the levels of intestinal bacteria (without changing the diet) can cause us to become overweight. Scientists bred genetically identical mice and split them into two groups. One group was given the intestinal bacteria from an obese person and the other group was given the bacteria from that person's lean twin. The two groups of mice were kept on the same diet, eating the same amount as each other, but the mice that got the bacteria from the obese person became overweight and had more body fat than the mice given the bacteria from the lean person.[161]

From this we can conclude that when good bacteria are in balance, we are less susceptible to weight gain and insulin resistance, which in turn protects our brain function.

If you need to take an antibiotic for an infection, take a probiotic throughout the course of antibiotics and for three months afterwards (take the probiotic and antibiotic at different times of day). If you are on a medication that reduces your beneficial bacteria on a continual basis, such as HRT, you might benefit from taking a probiotic all the time.

Avoid probiotic drinks, which often have high amounts of added sugar, and choose a probiotic that contains both *lactobacillus* and *bifidobacterium* strains (about 22 billion in total), as well as a prebiotic if possible (see NHP's Advanced Probiotic Support).

Testing probiotic levels

You can have a stool test – either through my clinic or by post – to assess your levels of beneficial bacteria. The test not only shows your levels of 'good' bacteria, but highlights if there are unhealthy negative bacteria living in your gut. It also flags up whether you have any yeasts like *candida*, or any parasites, and it tells you whether you are digesting and absorbing your food properly (see Resources Page 172 for information).

What to choose: probiotics

Avoid probiotic drinks. These can be high in sugar. Instead, go for a supplement that does not contain maltodextrin (which is rapidly converted to glucose and has a high GI of 110 and can affect blood sugar levels). Research suggests that maltodextrin can make you more prone to inflammation.[162] Also, probiotic drinks need a preservative to prolong their shelf life, usually in the form of potassium sorbate. A freeze-dried probiotic doesn't need a preservative or refrigerating, and it's easier to take it with you to protect your gut health wherever you go.

Mushroom supplements

The humble mushroom has been used for centuries for its medicinal benefits and for brain health. By far the best way to harness those benefits is in supplement form.

There are many varieties of mushroom, but the one most closely researched in terms of brain health is Lion's Mane *(Hericium erinaceus)*. In mice, this mushroom prevented spatial, short-term and visual recognition memory impairment that had been induced by beta-amyloid plaque build-up.[163] In human research, those taking a supplement of this mushroom showed improvement in mild cognitive impairment.[164]

Ongoing research suggests that Lion's Mane mushroom supplements could have anti-inflammatory and antioxidant properties, and could stimulate neuron regeneration and have neuroprotective effects.[165] The supplement appears to reduce the amount of beta-amyloid plaque build-up in the cerebral cortexes and hippocampi of Alzheimer's mice. Researchers suggest that this mushroom 'may have therapeutic potential for treating Alzheimer's as well as the other neurodegenerative diseases'.[166]

Herbs and spices

Cultures all over the world have used the medicinal properties of plants for hundreds of years – and I think it is very interesting that two of the licensed drugs for Alzheimer's are based on plants. Acetylcholinesterase inhibitors (see p.57) contain galantamine, which actually comes from the snowdrop; while rivastigmine comes from the calabar bean (an African legume). More plants are now being looked at as possible therapies for Alzheimer's.

Ginkgo biloba

This herb has been used since time immemorial to improve memory function, but it's also believed to improve the circulation, making it useful in the treatment of vascular dementia, as well as Alzheimer's. Ginkgo dilates the blood vessels, increasing blood flow to the brain, so helping to improve memory and concentration. It also functions as a powerful antioxidant, helping to fight free radical damage in the body. Research suggests that 'Ginkgo biloba is potentially beneficial for the improvement of cognitive function, activities of daily living, and global clinical assessment in patients with mild cognitive impairment or Alzheimer's disease.'[167]

Turmeric

Turmeric contains the compound curcumin, which has anti-inflammatory and antioxidant effects on the body. We know that controlling inflammation is important in the treatment of both dementia and Alzheimer's, and recent research suggests that curcumin 'possesses neuroprotective and cognitive-enhancing properties that may help delay or prevent neurodegenerative diseases, including Alzheimer's disease.'[168] As well as its anti-inflammatory and antioxidant effects, curcumin is thought to be able to inhibit beta-amyloid clumping.

Other herbs

Researchers looking at the effects of different herbs on memory and alertness have also been studying peppermint, chamomile and rosemary.

In one study, volunteers were asked to drink either a chamomile or peppermint tea and a control group were given hot water. The peppermint tea helped to improve long-term memory, working memory and alertness. As chamomile tea is known for its calming and sedative effects, it wasn't too much of a surprise then that it actually slowed down memory and attention speed.[169]

Scientists are investigating whether rosemary could help with brain health, studying a group of about 1,000 people who live in Acciaroli in Italy. About 300 of this group are centenarians and are free of both Alzheimer's and heart disease. They do eat a Mediterranean diet, but the scientists want to know why they have such a high level of older people free of disease.

One of the reasons could be that they use a lot of rosemary, because it grows abundantly in the area. A compound, called 1,8-cineole, in rosemary can boost levels of acetylcholine and could act in a similar way to the drugs licensed to treat Alzheimer's. This hypothesis is certainly borne out in studies on animals, which show that rosemary can improve memory[170] and increase the amount of antioxidant activity in the brain,[171] particularly in the hippocampus (the area responsible for memory).

> ## Give a sniff
>
> Interestingly, just smelling rosemary essential oils can make a difference to your memory. A study at Northumbria University, UK, tested whether putting people in a room scented with rosemary (compared to one scented with lavender and one with no scent at all) could make a difference to their ability to remember to do certain tasks. The researchers found that those in the rosemary-scented room had significantly enhanced prospective memory with scores 15 per cent higher than those in the room with no scent. They were also more alert. The lavender-scented room increased feelings of calmness and contentedness, but the volunteers had a decrease in their ability to remember to do the tasks at a given time – maybe it made them feel too laid back![172]

How to choose a good food supplement

When it comes to choosing supplements, you really do get what you pay for. So, while deciding which supplements to choose can be a minefield, as a rule of thumb always choose the most expensive you can afford. Other than that, and as well as the specific advice given for some of the supplements above, here are some general tips to help you differentiate the best from the rest.

Always choose capsules instead of tablets

Your digestive system has to work harder to release the nutrients from a tablet because it has to break down the binders that have been used to compress the ingredients into a solid shape, and the binders themselves are substances you're aiming to avoid in your foods, including sucrose, lactose, sugar alcohols (such as sorbitol) or synthetic polymers (such as polyethylene glycol). In comparison, with a capsule, your digestive system just has to dissolve the capsule in order to release the nutrients.

Choose vegetarian

If a supplement just says gelatine capsules then the gelatine is made from cow or pig gelatine, which is produced by boiling skin, ligaments, tendons or bones of the animal. I believe that vegetarian gelatine is a healthier option.

The exception is omega 3 fish oil supplements, which should come in capsules made from fish gelatine (it will be clear on the packaging that this is the case, if so).

Read the ingredients

While I hope it becomes second nature for you to read the labels on the food you buy, I also hope you'll stop to read the labels on the supplements you choose, too.

Perhaps surprisingly, many supplements contain additional ingredients that should be on the avoid list of anyone concerned about dementia and Alzheimer's. The ingredient list on supplements is just as important as the ingredients list on a packaged food – you may struggle to find it, though, as many manufacturers put it on the bottom of the box.

As with food, don't let the hype on the front or a long list of impressive-sounding ingredients or nutrients seduce you. What else has gone into to this supplement? There could be added sugar (remember that it may appear as glucose or fructose or another name for sugar), artificial sweeteners, colourings or flavourings. Chewable supplements may have other things added and effervescent tablets can contain high amounts of sodium bicarbonate which make them fizz and dissolve. Sodium has been linked to high blood pressure so it is better to avoid effervescent tablets.

Capsules often contain excipients, which are non-active ingredients with no nutritional value to you. Lubricants, anti-caking agents, disintegrants, fillers and bulking agents are all excipients. You may see them listed as magnesium stearate, titanium dioxide, talc, calcium hydrogen phosphate dehydrate and stearic acid. They make the supplements faster and easier to manufacture, saving the supplement producers time and money, but doing nothing for your nutritional health.

Without lubricants and anti-caking agents the manufacturing process has to be slowed down to allow the nutrients to flow into the capsules. This means that less heat is generated and this is beneficial when dealing with natural ingredients like herbs and enzymes. Furthermore, adding excipients means there is less space in each capsule – and seeing as companies are not required to list the amounts of excipient they have included in their product, you can't really be sure what proportion of active nutrient (compared with non-active ingredients) you're getting. The advice is simple: aim to choose just the vitamins and minerals – nothing more!

Look at the form of the nutrients

Your body absorbs different forms of the same nutrients in different ways. For example, not all calcium supplements are the same (see below). The form in which you take a nutrient supplement determines how well you absorb it and how effective it will be.

- Avoid inorganic mineral supplements. Oxides, sulphates, chlorides and carbonates are inorganic supplement forms (meaning they are geological forms – they come from the ground), which your body finds difficult to absorb and use compared with organic mineral supplements that come from plants. For example, if you have ever taken iron as ferrous sulphate, you'll know that it can cause black stools or constipation. This is because ferrous sulphate is an inorganic form of iron and your body absorbs only about 2–10 per cent of the iron in the supplement. The remainder is flushed through your bowels.

- Choose mineral supplements in their organic forms. Citrates and ascorbates are examples of organic forms of mineral. For example, calcium in the form of calcium ascorbate is almost 30 per cent more absorbable than calcium carbonate; likewise magnesium taken as magnesium citrate (300mg of magnesium in the form of inorganic magnesium oxide gives only around 6 per cent absorption; whereas as magnesium citrate you absorb up to 90 per cent of the supplement). This pattern is replicated for all mineral supplements.

Chapter 9

Step 3: Exercise

We all know that exercise is important for our general health, including the health of our heart, blood pressure, blood sugar balance, mood, digestion and bones. However, it is also important for mental and cognitive health – not only does it promote feel-good factors, but (along with a healthy, well-balanced diet) it helps prevent weight gain.

You will know that it is important for your general health and wellbeing that you are not overweight but it is just as important specifically for your brain function. Your brain could age ten years faster if you are overweight when you are middle aged, compared with someone of a normal weight at that age.[173]

Brain scans on people aged between 20 and 87 showed that the people who were overweight at middle age had changes in their brain structure that would only normally be seen in people much older. The volume of white matter that connects different areas of the brain had shrunk much more if the person's BMI (Body Mass Index; the ratio of weight to height) was above 25. This accelerated shrinkage was seen only from middle age onwards, so the 50-year-old overweight person had a brain that looked like a 60-year-old's brain. The conclusion was that your brain may be more vulnerable to being overweight in middle age than in your youth. The researchers have suggested that this could be owing to the fact that fat cells cause inflammation, which we already know is a risk factor for both vascular dementia and Alzheimer's.

However, although the study used BMI as the marker for healthy (or unhealthy) weight, I don't think it is a good measure.

Body Mass Index (BMI) versus Body Fat Percentage (BFP)

BMI is calculated by dividing your weight in kilograms by the square of your height in metres.

For example, if your weight is 63.5kg and your height is 1.68m, your BMI = 63.5 divided by (1.68x1.68) = 22.5. In order to assess your relative health with regards to your weight, you apply this figure to the following scale:

A BMI of 20 to 25 is normal.

A BMI of 25 to 30 indicates you are overweight.

A BMI of 30 to 40 indicates you are obese.

A BMI of 40 or more indicates you are dangerously obese (that is, your weight is posing a severe risk to your health).

However, BMI cannot distinguish between fat and muscle and we know that, in fact, muscle is heavier than fat. So, a very fit athlete who has a high BMI but very low BFP might tip into the overweight category on the BMI scale, even though their weight is mostly down to muscle. A sedentary person with the same BMI as the athlete might a very high BFP and be considerably less fit and healthy.

It's now possible to measure a person's total body fat using a special machine that looks like a set of bathrooms scales. It passes an electrical current through the body, measuring the speed at which the current moves. Because muscle is a far better electricity conductor than fat, the faster the current moves through the body, the greater the proportion of muscle compared with fat. The results are given as a percentage of total body fat.

Where your fat is located on your body is also important. I wrote a best-selling book a few years ago called *Fat Around the Middle*. We know that carrying more weight around the middle of your body increases your risk of type 2 diabetes and heart disease. Interesting research has shown that if you have fat around your middle when you are middle aged, you increase your risk of developing dementia or Alzheimer's *thirty years later*. This risk exists whether or not you have type 2 diabetes or heart problems.[174] Up to 50 per cent of adults carry fat around the middle, so it is important to make dietary and lifestyle changes as soon as you can to reduce your waistline.

To calculate if you are carrying too much fat around your middle, do these simple measurements:

1. Measure your waist in centimetres, finding where it is the narrowest.

2. Measure your hips in centimetres at their widest point.

3. Divide your waist measurement by your hip measurement to calculate your ratio. For example: 79cm waist divided by 94cm hip = 0.84

If the ratio of your waist-to-hip measurement is more than 0.8 for women and 0.95 for men, you may have a greater risk of Alzheimer's. You may also have an increased risk of heart disease, type 2 diabetes, high blood pressure and cancer (and especially breast cancer).

How much exercise is enough?

Just 30 minutes of exercise, three days a week for four weeks can have an impact. In one study, subjects were asked to spend their 30 minutes using a combination exercise programme that included aerobics, strength training and stretching. Those who followed the programme showed improvements in memory and processing speed, compared with those who did not.[175] Interestingly, the combined approach to exercise seems to have a greater effect than just aerobic exercises alone for improving cognitive function.[176]

In another study, yoga has been shown to be more effective at improving memory than brain training.[177] In the study, people over the age of 55 who had problems with their memory, including not being able to remember faces and names, were split into two groups. One group was given one hour's brain training a week, while the other practised one hour of yoga a week and meditation for 20 minutes a day. Both brain training and yoga improve verbal memory, but the yoga had the added benefit of improving visual–spatial memory, too. This is the memory that helps with remembering locations.

Researchers hypothesise that the positive effects of exercise on cognitive function occur because exercise can increase hippocampal volume by 2 per cent, reversing age-related loss in volume by one to two years.[178] (The hippocampus is the part of the brain that shrinks as a symptom of Alzheimer's.)

In the researchers' words the findings 'indicate that aerobic exercise training is effective at reversing hippocampal volume loss in late adulthood, which is accompanied by improved memory function'.

Keep sexually active

A huge study (entitled 'Sex on the Brain!') of more than 6,800 people aged 50 to 89 showed that those who were still active in the bedroom had sharper cognitive function. Men who were sexually active scored higher by 23 per cent on word tests and 3 per cent on number puzzles. Women scored higher by 14 per cent on word tests and 2 per cent on number puzzles. It is thought that the benefit could come from the release of neurotransmitters such as dopamine into the brain during sex.[179]

Chapter 10

Step 4: Stress and sleep

Midlife stress may increase your risk of Alzheimer's and other forms of dementia, according to a study of 800 women living in Sweden, whose wellbeing was assessed for nearly four decades. The study began in 1968 when the women were in their 40s or 50s, and, over the next 38 years, they were given regular health assessments every five to ten years.[180] At the beginning of the study, the women were asked whether they had experienced major stresses such as divorce, the death of a spouse or child, or serious illness in a close family member. Other sources of stress they were asked about included their own or their partner's unemployment, a lack of social support or a history of abuse.

At each follow-up visit, the women were also asked whether they had experienced symptoms of stress lasting at least a month. Such symptoms included irritability, feeling tense or fearful, nervousness, anxiety or sleeping poorly. The more stressful events they had experienced in the past, the more likely they were to experience symptoms of distress.

At the start of the study, about 25 per cent of the women had experienced one major, stressful life event, 23 per cent had experienced at least two, 20 per cent had experienced at least three, and 16 per cent had experienced four or more. The most common major stressor was mental illness in a close family member.

During the follow-up period, over the next four decades, around one in five of the women had developed dementia, most often Alzheimer's, at an average age of 78. Those who reported experiencing the most stressful events in middle age were at 21 per cent increased risk of developing Alzheimer's in old age, and at 15 per cent higher risk of developing other forms of dementia.

This all tells us that controlling our stress levels is crucial for minimising our risk of developing dementia.

Types of stress

There are two types of stress: short term (acute) when you, say, ride a rollercoaster; and long-term (chronic) stress, which is most harmful to your health.

Long-term stress is often triggered by serious life events. Financial downturn, bereavement, work pressures and family trauma can all begin the stress response. However, although there may be a significant event that provides the trigger, when stress is ongoing, long-term and therefore chronic, the feeling of it may become so normal to you that you are not actually aware that stress is there. Therefore, it's useful to be aware of the symptoms of chronic stress. These include:

- Sleep problems
- Back, neck and head pain from tense muscles
- Digestive disorders
- Hair loss
- Fatigue
- High blood pressure
- Palpitations
- Chest pain
- Skin problems (hives, eczema and other rashes)
- Jaw pain (from grinding your teeth)
- Sexual difficulties
- Recurrent colds and infections
- Nervousness, anxiety and panic attacks
- Depression and moodiness
- Irritability and frustration
- Memory problems and lack of concentration

Try to devise strategies to reduce the amount of stress you are under – asking for help, delegating, and learning to say no are all good ways to start. If your job is stressing you a lot, can you change it – if not completely, then in small but significant ways (reduce your hours, move department, work from home for part of the week)? If friends are overloading you, can you take a step back? Without positive action, no treatment plan will be as effective as it could be.

You may conclude that you can't control the stress – but you can control how it affects you physically, and you can make sure you are not exacerbating it. There is a chance that your pattern of eating is subconsciously telling your body that it is under even more stress. That's because, if your blood-sugar levels fluctuate, your body releases adrenaline, which is the same hormone it releases when you are under stress.

Try to keep your blood-sugar levels and energy levels stable by eating something every three hours. Eat breakfast, lunch and dinner, plus a snack mid-morning and one mid-afternoon, with no longer than three hours between. This will stop those roller-coaster highs and lows and cravings for sweet foods. Because your blood sugar isn't allowed to drop, your body will no longer have to ask you for a quick fix. As your blood sugar steadies, so will your mood swings. And as your adrenaline levels reduce, you will automatically start to feel happier and calmer inside.

Some nutrients have a special role to play in helping to reduce stress levels. When you are under stress you use up a lot of your B vitamins – especially vitamins B2 and B5 – as well as vitamin C. These are all water-soluble vitamins, so your need to eat them in your diet on a day-to-day basis (or get them from food supplements), because your body doesn't store them. The best sources of all the B vitamins are whole grains, green leafy vegetables, and nuts and seeds.

The other nutrient that prolonged stress depletes is magnesium, a calming mineral often referred to as 'Nature's tranquilliser'. It helps to relieve anxiety and relax muscles. One common symptom of magnesium deficiency is waking up in the early hours of the morning and not being able to get back to sleep. Increase your intake of green leafy vegetables, nuts and seeds to boost your magnesium levels.

Supplements to combat stress

As well as magnesium and B vitamins, there are other supplements that are good for restoring equilibrium to your sense of calm.

- **Siberian ginseng.** This regulates the production of cortisol and acts as a tonic to your adrenal glands. It is an adaptogen, which means it can help your body to adapt in any way it needs in order to cope with stress. It also helps with energy levels, stamina and endurance – and it can boost immunity, too.

- **L-theanine.** This amino acid is found in some green teas. It helps transmit nerve impulses in the brain and reduces stress and anxiety.

- **Rhodiola.** Another adaptogenic herb which works in the same way as Siberian ginseng.

In my clinic I use NHP's Tranquil Woman Support, which contains Siberian ginseng, l-theanine, magnesium, aloe vera, B vitamins (plus extra B5), chromium and turmeric (see www.naturalhealthpractice. com). Although it is called 'Tranquil Woman', this supplement is just as good for men as none of the ingredients are gender specific.

Meditation and mindfulness

Studies show that meditation can not only help relieve stress, but also improve brain function. In one study, researchers took a group of adults between the ages of 55 and 90 with Mild Cognitive Impairment (MCI, which can lead to dementia in about 50 per cent of cases) and asked them to practise a guided meditation for 15 to 30 minutes a day for eight weeks, as well as attend weekly mindfulness check-ins.[181]

Eight weeks later, MRI scans showed improved functional connectivity in the default mode network (the part of your brain that never shuts down) and slowed shrinkage of the hippocampus, the main part of the brain responsible for memory that usually shrinks with dementia. Participants also showed an overall improvement in cognition and wellbeing.

Links with sleep

When you're stressed you produce the hormones adrenaline and cortisol. Cortisol has a circadian rhythm, meaning that its levels fluctuate over the course of 24 hours. Levels should be highest when you wake in the morning, revving you up ready to start the day, and then lower when you go to sleep and lowest of all during the night.

Cortisol is almost the direct opposite of another hormone, melatonin. Levels of melatonin are highest at night and then fall off to their lowest levels by the morning. However, if you are stressed and your cortisol levels stay high, melatonin production stays low, making it hard for you to go to sleep.

Too little sleep increases your risk for Alzheimer's because beta-amyloid protein is cleared away during sleep when your cerebrospinal fluid washes out toxins from your body.

Interestingly, research on mice has shown that the cerebrospinal detoxification process happens only when a mouse is sleeping. As soon as the mouse goes to sleep, the cerebrospinal fluid floods through the brain. At the same time brain cells seem to shrink, making space for the fluid to flow freely through and around them clearing out the waste This process does not happen when the mouse is awake.

So what happens if you're not sleeping well? We know that in mice who have been bred to model Alzheimer's, sleep deprivation causes a substantial increase in beta-amyloid plaque build-up.[182] And when researchers have looked at older people without Alzheimer's, those who are sleeping for shorter amounts of time and have poor-quality sleep have more beta-amyloid plaque build-up.[183]

Getting good amounts of good-quality sleep is crucial (aim for six to eight hours uninterrupted sleep every night). And the position in which you sleep can also be a factor. When you sleep on your side, your body seems more able to remove the build-up of so-called 'brain waste' chemicals, such as beta-amyloid proteins, that are thought to contribute to this and other neurological diseases such as Parkinson's.[184]

If you are not already sleeping well, you should look at your bedtime routine. Poor 'sleep hygiene' is the most common cause of insomnia and disturbed sleep. Your busy, active brain needs to be treated like a dimmer switch and allowed to wind down slowly. Ideally, you should allow about 40 minutes to switch off with whatever relaxing routine you find most helpful – for example, having a bath, reading, or listening to an audio book. But before you do any of that, you need to switch off your TV, phone and tablet – at least an hour (ideally two) before you intend to go to bed. This is not just about bombarding your brain with information just before you try to sleep, there are physical factors at work: backlit screens, such as those of a tablet or smartphone, emit blue light that interferes with your body's production of melatonin – the hormone that regulates your body's circadian rhythm, the 24-hour rhythm of day and night.[185] As it goes, exposure to bright light of any colour before bed will suppress your melatonin production – it's just that blue light is worst of all. Studies show that sitting in bright light compared to a dim light delays melatonin onset and shortens melatonin exposure by up to 90 minutes – that is, it takes a full hour and a half for the effects of bright-light exposure to wear off and melatonin to kick in and make you feel sleepy. If the room light is left on during sleep, melatonin secretion is suppressed by greater than 50 per cent.[186]

Unsurprisingly, then, researchers suggest that 'chronically exposing oneself to electrical lighting in the late evening disrupts melatonin signalling and could therefore potentially impact [not only] sleep, [but also] thermoregulation [our ability to control our temperature], blood pressure, and glucose homeostasis.' Interestingly, in a direct link with brain health, in experiments using mice, melatonin has been shown to reduce the levels of beta-amyloid protein in the brain and to help flush it out.[187]

Top tips for a good night's sleep

As well as putting away screens one to two hours before you go to bed and creating a relaxing bedtime routine, try adopting the following as part of your good sleep hygiene:

- Use blackout curtains or blinds, which can stop morning light waking you too early and will help to mask the light of bright street light, if you have it, outside your bedroom window.

- Don't have an alarm clock or night light that emits a light during the night.

- If you need a night light (for example, to light your way to the loo), then use a dim, red light, as this bypasses your optic nerves in such a way as not to interfere with your body's production of melatonin.

- Get lots of bright light during the day and early evening, as this will help improve your sleep and melatonin levels.[188] It could also help prevent sundowning (an increased state of confusion towards the end of the day) in people with Alzheimer's.

- Keep your bedroom cooler rather than warmer, then layer on blankets that you can add or remove during the night if you get too cold or hot.

- Use cotton bedding, which will enable your body to regulate your temperature more effectively during the night, improving your ability to sleep through.

- Get a comfortable mattress – the best and most comfortable you can afford!

Then, try these other natural solutions to better sleep:

- Take vitamin C to keep your stress hormones in check (see p.117).

- Take probiotics to help your body produce serotonin (vital for making the hormone melatonin; see above).

- Add in magnesium and lemon balm to help relax your body.

- Try tinctures of the herbs valerian and passionflower, which can influence certain brain chemicals to to calm your mind and help you relax.

- Try homeopathy. Opt for *Chamomilla* if you're feeling tired, but can't get off to sleep; *Cocculus* for insomnia caused by mental and physical exhaustion; *Coffea* if you've too many thoughts running through your head; or *arnica* if you're overtired and restless.

- Use aromatherapy. spritz your pillow with lavender or melissa, or massage one or other of these oils (check for suitable dilutions, as necessary) into your temples and pulse points.

Melatonin supplementation

As we've already seen (see p.136), the function of melatonin is crucial for a good night's sleep and even may have a direct impact on the progression of Alzheimer's itself. So, wouldn't it be wonderful if we could take it as a supplement?

Melatonin used to be available in tablets in health food shops in the UK (and in the USA it still is), but I would not recommend using it without medical supervision: it is a hormone, not a nutrient, so I believe it should be prescribed by a medical practitioner. Taking one hormone is likely to affect the balance of other hormones in your system, because your hormones work in a feedback loop – one triggering changes in the levels of another to make up your whole endocrine system. I believe it's much better to address the underlying causes of your sleep problems (whether they are a result of stress, poor sleep hygiene or another cause), so that you restore balance throughout your body, as well as restoring good sleep. Furthermore, melatonin supplementation comes with side-effects, including daytime sleepiness, headaches, dizziness, irritability, depression and stomach cramps. Melatonin might also increase blood glucose (sugar) levels, so people with diabetes would have to be extra careful and, anyway, when we're aiming to reduce the risk of Alzheimer's balanced sugar levels are key.

Acupuncture

This traditional Chinese treatment can be used to treat sleep problems – but it may also help people to retain their memory as they get older and may even delay cognitive decline in the early stages of dementia.[189] There is not much published research on acupuncture and dementia, but the suggestion is that it could improve scores on cognitive tests and may be particularly helpful when used alongside dementia drugs.

Chapter 11

Step 5: Your environment

How you look after your body in terms of how you nourish it, how you keep it working physically and how well you rest it are all crucial to maintaining your cognitive health for as long as possible. The environment in which you live and function is important, too. (Remember the section on epigenetics in Chapter 4– your environment will influence your health and that of future generations of your family.)

We are all exposed to environmental toxins and pollutants, and the impact of toxins on your body and your brain function is partly dependent on how well you eat and how well your body functions. Nutrients such as probiotics, which help flush out toxins from your gut, can help improve your detoxification processes, but you also need to make sure your liver – your main organ of detoxification, your inbuilt waste-disposal unit – is working efficiently.

Nourish your liver

Your liver is the largest organ in your body (not counting the skin), with tremendous powers of regeneration. You can cut your liver in half and it will regrow. Seeing as its cells are replaced every five months, you can easily improve the way your liver works. Artichokes and dandelion greens help your liver produce the bile it needs to break fats into small molecules that your body can digest; onions, leeks and garlic contain sulphur compounds that are important for efficient liver function, as do cruciferous vegetables, such as cabbage, cauliflower and broccoli. Supplements of magnesium and B vitamins are also important for good liver function.

If those are the foods and nutrients you should increase in your diet, those that you should avoid begin with alcohol. Classed as a hepatoxin, alcohol is unequivocally toxic for your liver.

Your body can break down alcohol at the rate of one unit an hour. However, if your rate of alcohol consumption exceeds that at any given moment, your liver becomes overloaded. It can't break down the alcohol fast enough to eliminate it, and over time this can result in fatty liver disease.

So, look after your liver by nourishing it well, but also do your best to avoid the toxins that can make it work too hard.

Avoid heavy metals

Toxic metals can affect you in two ways. First, they have a directly toxic effect that can cause damage to your tissues. Second, they can interfere with important nutrients that you need for good health, which results in nutrient deficiency.

Aluminium

You probably have heard that aluminium exposure can increase the risk of a person developing Alzheimer's but, even after decades of research, there is still a lot of controversy around the subject.

Aluminium is commonly found in cookware, kitchen foil, deodorants and antiperspirants. It also occurs in antacid medication and is an anti-caking agent in dried milk and other foods, such as baking powder. It can occur naturally in our water supply.

Some studies show higher levels of aluminium in the brains of people with Alzheimer's.[190] The Alzheimer's Society UK says 'Current medical and scientific opinion of the relevant research indicates that the findings do not convincingly demonstrate a causal relationship between aluminium and Alzheimer's disease.' So, even though higher levels of aluminium can be found in the brains of people with Alzheimer's, we don't yet know which comes first – is it that high levels of aluminium in the brain cause Alzheimer's, or is it that Alzheimer's causes a build-up of aluminium in the brain?

Nonetheless, some scientists are much more vocal about the negative effects of aluminium. Findings from a study reviewed in 2016 say that 'Aluminium is a widely recognised neurotoxin.'[191]

It is known to cause the accumulation of tau protein and beta-amyloid in experimental animals.[192] And a scientific paper published 2011 asks the question 'Aluminium and Alzheimer's disease: after a century of controversy, is there a plausible link?'[193] This paper puts forward some interesting points. It says that the link between aluminium and Alzheimer's has been disputed because:

- Aluminium cannot enter the brain in sufficient amounts to cause damage.

- Excess aluminium is efficiently excreted from the body.

- Aluminium accumulation in neurons is a consequence rather than a cause of neuronal loss.

But the author counters these arguments by saying:

- Very small amounts of aluminium are needed to produce neurotoxicity.

- Aluminium has a way of passing through the brain barrier.

- Small amounts of aluminium over a lifetime of exposure can cause accumulation in brain tissue.

'The hypothesis that aluminium significantly contributes to Alzheimer's is built upon very solid experimental evidence and should not be dismissed. Immediate steps should be taken to lessen human exposure to aluminium, which may be the single most aggravating and avoidable factor related to Alzheimer's disease.'

I believe that it is much better then to err on the side of caution, limiting your exposure to aluminium as much as possible. As a start, throw out any aluminium-based cookware and replace it with cast iron, enamel, glass and stainless steel. Check ingredients lists of foods for added aluminium and buy aluminium-free baking powder and aluminium-free deodorant.

Mercury

Classed as a neurotoxin, mercury is thought to pose an increased risk of developing Alzheimer's.[194] The saying 'mad as a hatter' refers to the traditional practice of polishing top hats with mercury –

which could lead to mercury poisoning! We may not wear top hats so much anymore, but you will still find mercury in some dental amalgams and some fish.

But, before you decide to strip fish from your diet, recent research has shown that even though eating seafood once a week is associated with higher levels of mercury in the brain, there is less Alzheimer's disease in those people eating the seafood – so the overall impact of eating seafood once a week is positive.[195] The researchers analysed the autopsied brains of 286 people who had participated in a study that asked them to keep food diaries for up to 4.5 years before their death (the average age when they died was 90). The brain mercury levels reflected the number of seafood meals they consumed each week, so the more seafood they ate, the higher the level of mercury. However, the researchers found that those who were eating seafood at least once a week had less Alzheimer's disease in the brain with less beta-amyloid plaque build-up, and a reduced spread of neurofibrillary tangles.

Although seafood can contain mercury, it also contains good amount of selenium – a mineral known to reduce mercury toxicity. In an editorial in the same edition of this research, academics from Canada stated that this report provides 'reassurance that seafood contamination with mercury is not related to increased brain pathology'. And that 'Eating fatty fish may continue to be considered potentially beneficial against cognitive decline in at least a proportion of older adults, a strategy that now generally should not be affected by concerns about mercury contamination in fish.'[196]

If you want to keep your mercury levels lower, avoid shark, swordfish and marlin. These larger fish can contain proportionally higher levels of mercury because they feed off smaller fish that are already contaminated. Canned tuna contains less mercury than fresh tuna, because the fish used for canning is younger, with less accumulated mercury, than the fish that we buy fresh. But canned tuna also contains lower levels of beneficial omega 3 fats.

If you have mercury amalgam fillings, consider replacing them at a specialist dentist who understands how to remove the toxic fillings safely. Once mercury fillings start to crack, they could be releasing mercury vapour – at which point changing them is essential.

Pesticides

There has been some research looking at the effects of pesticides on brain health because they can increase beta-amyloid levels. It has been found that higher blood levels of pesticides are found in people with Alzheimer's and it is thought that people with the APOE4 gene (which puts them more at risk of Alzheimer's; see p.45) may be more susceptible to the negative effects of pesticide exposure.[197] Some of the pesticides levels in the people with Alzheimer's were very high.

However, this research is based on findings in brains that had been exposed to the pesticide DDT, which has been banned for many years, suggesting that the exposure was very early on in the subjects' lives. It's hard to establish cause and effect because of the extended period of time between exposure and damage to cognitive function. (Research into the negative effects of smoking had the same problem, because it takes decades for lung disease to manifest itself, making it again difficult to connect cause and effect.)

However, other research has found lower cognitive performance in people who have been exposed to pesticides as a result of their job.[198] And even just environmental exposure to pesticides has been shown to increase the risk of Alzheimer's. A study involving more than 17,000 people showed that those who lived in areas with high pesticide use had an increased risk of Alzheimer's. The researchers said 'this study supports and extends previous findings and provides an indication that environmental exposure to pesticides may affect the human health by increasing the incidence of certain neurological disorders at the level of the general population.'[199]

The danger of pesticides is borne out in the behaviour of bees. Pesticides can affect the bees' brain nerve cells, causing epilepsy-like brain activity and then shutting down their learning centres.[200] The result has been a dramatic decline in bee population.

So what's in pesticides that's causing the problems in humans? Organophosphates, which are the basis of many pesticides, reduce levels of acetylcholine (which is important for memory and learning) and this may be the reason that pesticides can increase the risk of Alzheimer's.

Try to limit your exposure to pesticides where you can, especially if you are a keen gardener. Buy organic food, which has not been treated with pesticides, and always wash and peel any non-organic produce before you eat it.

Diesel fumes

Diesel engines emit tiny particles that have been found in the brains of people who have suffered neurodegenerative disease, including Alzheimer's. Called magnetite, these tiny particles were originally thought to have occurred naturally,[201] but now we think that they can travel into the brain, triggering cognitive malfunction. Magnetite is also linked to free radical production (see p.83).

When scientists analysed the particles, they found that they had a fused surface suggesting that they had been formed under extreme heat – as in a car engine.[202] As well as diesel engines, which emit up to 22 times more of these particles than petrol engines, the particles can also be released by open fires, stoves and the powders in photocopier toners.

Endocrine Disrupting Chemicals (EDCs)

EDCs are a widespread environmental toxin. They mostly mimic the effects of hormones in the body, confusing your endocrine system. However, researchers now think that EDCs could have an effect on your brain function.[203] It used to be thought that the connections in our brains were fixed and that we couldn't do anything to change that. But we now know that this is not the case and that the connections have the ability to change in response to learning. This is the concept of neuroplasticity – it's the reason why learning a second language can help with brain health because language learning forms different pathways and connections in the brain.

This plasticity – the ability to generate new nerve cells and neural structures – is there no matter what age you are. The concern is that EDCs (as well as heavy metals) may impair it.

EDCs are found in plastics, pesticides, hormone medications (like the Pill and HRT), water supply, dental fillings, till and credit-card receipts, the white resins coating the inside of food and drink cans, toiletries, cosmetics, lipsticks, perfumes, hair spray, nail polish, toothpaste, spermicides, deodorants and body washes.

One EDC is bisphenol A (BPA), which is used in the manufacture of plastics. Investigations into the neurotoxicity of BPA have shown that it seems to have effects on the brain similar to those seen in Alzheimer's and may cause cognitive decline.[204]

To reduce your exposure to BPA:

- Don't rinse out plastic bottles or containers in very hot water as BPA leeches out 55 times faster than normal in hot water.

- Buy BPA-free plastic bottles.

- Be careful of takeaway hot drinks in plastic cups, because chemicals will leech out quickly from the plastic.

- Reduce the amount of canned foods and drinks you consume, because of the plastic coating inside the cans.

- If your job requires you to handle thermal paper (tickets or credit-card receipts), wash your hands regularly.

- Avoid food that needs to be microwaved in a plastic container as the plastic can break down in the high temperatures, releasing the chemicals.

- Don't leave plastic water bottles sitting in direct sunlight on a window sill or in the car.

- Look for the code at the bottom of plastic containers. Some plastics that are marked with recycle codes 3 or 7 may be made from BPA.[205] Avoid these.

Nobody really knows the long-term effects of EDCs and particularly the cocktail effect of a number of EDCs mixed together. In clinical trials, researchers look at the toxic effect of one chemical at a time. In order to do your best to protect yourself against any harmful effects, look at the following list and try to avoid them in the cleaning products, toiletries and fragrances you use around your home.

- Parabens (such as methylparabens)
- Phthalates
- Talc
- Triclosan
- Surfactants
- Synthetic fragrances (parfum)
- Formaldehyde
- BHT

- DEA, MEA, TEA
- Polyethylene glycol
- Propylene glycol
- Sodium lauryl (laureth) sulphate
- Colourants
- Petrochemicals
- Urea
- Butylphenyl Methylpropional

Smoking and alcohol

Two considerable sources of stress on the liver are toxins that, by and large, we can control – those in cigarettes and alcohol.

Smoking

Just under one in five (19 per cent) of adults in Great Britain now smoke: 20 per cent of men and 17 per cent of women – about 9.6 million adult smokers in all. Research shows that smokers are twice as likely to develop Alzheimer's and vascular dementia as non-smokers. The good news is that smoking rates have halved since 1974, when 51 per cent of men and 41 per cent of women smoked. Surveys show that about two-thirds of current smokers would like to stop, although only 30 to 40 per cent attempt to do so in a given year. Studies show that if you do stop smoking, your risks of developing smoking-related illnesses reduce with every day, week, month and year that you remain a non-smoker. The positive effects on your circulation and blood pressure begin from the moment you quit.

What works for you will depend entirely on the nature of your own addiction and your commitment to quitting. If you smoke to control your weight, try something weight-loss-centred, such as replacing the cigarette with a stick of celery. It's nutritious, will fill a hunger gap and has almost zero calories. Holding it and munching on it will give your hands and mouth something to do until your cigarette craving has passed. Eventually you'll break free of the addiction – and won't have gained weight in the process!

You may find that nicotine replacement therapy (patches or gum) will work for you, but remember that nicotine is addictive and you still have to shake off that addiction. It is also a harmful chemical, shown to fuel some lung cancer cells if they are already present. Some of the best results I've seen have been as a result of hypnotherapy treatment – but acupuncture can be effective, too.

Alcohol

The government recommends drinking no more than 14 units of alcohol a week – whether you are a man or a woman. On top of that, it is best to drink no more than two units in one day (so no one recommends saving up the week's units for one, big night out!) However, statistics show that at least 9 million of us drink above these levels – a worrying risk factor for dementia.

Brain capacity naturally declines with age, but studies show that the brains of men who regularly drink alcohol appear between 1.5 to 5.7 years older than their lower-unit counterparts.[206] Many alcoholics who give up drinking continue to have a poorer memory and lower attention span and problem-solving skills for up to a year after they quit;[207] although cognitive function appears to take more than a year to get back to normal.

Drinking alcohol earlier in life may substantially increase the risks of developing early onset dementia (before the age of 65). People who heavily misuse alcohol also often suffer injuries to the head – from falls or fights – and have a poor diet, all of which can contribute to alcohol-related dementia.

Working out how many units you are consuming can be difficult.

For example, a large glass of wine (175ml) may be more than two units, depending on its abv (alcohol by volume). To work out your units, always check the abv of a drink. Multiply the total volume of a drink by its abv and divide the result by 1,000. For example, 175ml x 13% abv divided by 1,000 leaves you with 2.3. So that glass of wine is 2.3 units and it is already above the recommendation for your night's drinking.

Reducing your toxic load could have untold benefits for your brain – and even though the information in this chapter may seem alarming, especially if you realise you've been using some of the chemicals in your home for a long time, it's never too late to start removing them from your life. In being proactive you will feel in greater control of your health and that is always a good thing for your overall wellbeing.

Chapter 12

Step 6: Brain training

Can you protect your brain by exercising it in the same way that you exercise your body? And, if so, what kind of exercise should you be doing? Will Sudoku keep you thinking clearly – or just make you an expert at Sudoku? Is it possible for anyone to exercise their brain sufficiently – or is your mental capability something you were born with?

There are still many unanswered questions relating to the subject of brain training. But some clues came from a post-mortem study of 670 nuns' brains. This study compared the brains of the nuns with the symptoms they had displayed (or not) before death. What was interesting was that the nuns who had been accustomed to writing grammatically complex (so called 'high-density ideas') essays in earlier life (in their 20s) seemed to have avoided Alzheimer's in later life – at least they showed no outward signs of it. Meanwhile, all of those who had what the researchers called 'low-density ideas' in their writing were showing signs of the disease. However, when the brains were examined after death, some of those high-density-idea nuns who had shown no signs of Alzheimer's in life did in fact have signs of damage in their brains.[208]

So, what does this tell us? What seems to be the case is that using your brain may offset the damage that may be occurring inside, but it may not stave it off completely. Think about the novelist Iris Murdoch. In her last novel, written before she was diagnosed with Alzheimer's, her vocabulary had dwindled and become simpler, although her grammar remained complex, consistent with earlier work. It has since been said that the author's 26 novels provide a unique resource for studying the impact of Alzheimer's on the language system of the brain.

It is worth doing all you can to keep your brain active and healthy. There is the concept of 'brain or cognitive reserve': that brain function is not fixed but has a degree of plasticity. If you view your brain as a muscle, if you don't use it, it will atrophy. In the same way that you would exercise your muscles, if you exercise and stimulate your brain it could be possible to improve your brain reserve, stimulating your brain to form new connections.

Taking part in leisure activities such as reading, dancing, and playing board games and musical instruments has been shown to reduce the risk of dementia.[209] Research conducted over five years on people with an average age of 79 in the Bronx Ageing Study asked subjects how many cognitive activities they participated in (reading, writing, crossword puzzles, board or card games or playing music) and for how many days a week. An 'activity day' was classed as doing that activity for one day a week. They found that for every 'activity day' in which the subjects participated, they delayed the onset of rapid memory loss by two months. Those who took part in 11 activity days per month delayed the onset of dementia by 15.5 months.[210] So the more activities you do, and the more often you do them, the greater the benefits. Doing crosswords has been found to be particularly beneficial in delaying memory decline – by 2.5 years.[211]

Electronic brain games

In recent years, the advent of the brain-training computer programmes and apps has added a new dimension for research – that into how significantly electronic brain games might slow cognitive decline.

Results from a ten-year study called the ACTIVE study (Advanced Cognitive Training for Independent and Vital Elderly), which has been funded by the US National Institute on Ageing, has been looking at the effects of brain training on people with an average age of 73 at the start of the study.

A quarter of the people were not given any training at all. The remaining participants were divided into three groups.

For five weeks, each of the three groups was given ten one-hour training sessions. One group participated in classroom courses on techniques to improve memory; another was given classroom skills to improve reasoning; the third was given computerised training to increase the speed of visual processing, which is how you take in information from the cues you see (the speed with which you can do this naturally declines with age).

The people in the three groups who got the brain-training exercises had a 33 per cent lower risk of developing Alzheimer's than those who did not get any training at all. Furthermore, the research found that those in the computerised brain training group had a delayed decline in cognitive function compared with those in the other groups. So, electronic brain training not only reduced the decline, but also delayed its onset. The effect was there, but was less significant, in the classroom memory and reasoning groups.

Then, some of the computerised brain-training participants got some extra refresher classes 11 and 35 months after the initial sessions. For these people the risk of cognitive decline or dementia was reduced to 48 per cent.[212]

It's not all rosy

However, there has been a lot of criticism of the multimillion-pound industry that is computer-based brain training programmes and apps. In 2014, the Stanford Centre on Longevity consensus on the brain-training industry stated that the cognitive benefits of these games were 'frequently exaggerated and at times misleading'.[213] It says that 'brain games' are promoted to reassure and entice a worried public. The Stanford Centre on Longevity and the Berlin Max Planck Institute for Human Development put together a number of questions to ask the world's leading cognitive psychologists and neuroscientists in order to be able to give a consensus view on the subject. The questions they wanted answered were:

- What do expert scientists think about these claims and promises?

- Do they have specific recommendations for effective ways to boost cognition in healthy, older adults?

- Are there merits to the claimed benefits of the brain games and, if so, do older adults benefit from brain-game learning in the same ways younger people do?

- How large are the gains associated with computer-based cognitive exercises? Are the gains restricted to specific skills or does general cognitive aptitude improve?

- How does playing games compare with other proposed means of mitigating age-related declines, such as physical activity and exercise, meditation, or social engagement?

The summary of the consensus was:

'We object to the claim that brain games offer consumers a scientifically grounded avenue to reduce or reverse cognitive decline when there is no compelling scientific evidence to date that they do. The promise of a magic bullet detracts from the best evidence to date, which is that cognitive health in old age reflects the long-term effects of healthy, engaged lifestyles. In the judgment of the signatories, exaggerated and misleading claims exploit the anxiety of older adults about impending cognitive decline. We encourage continued careful research and validation in this field.'

They acknowledge that our brains remain malleable even as we get older (the concept of brain plasticity). They also accept that as we learn new skills or have new experiences, there can be an increase in the number of synapses and neurons and a strengthening of the connections between them. Their concern is really just a question of whether electronic brain-training games are better than any other skill that we can practise and learn.

Speaking a second language

Speaking a second language throughout your life could delay the onset of Alzheimer's. Studies show that people who speak two languages may develop dementia more than four years later than those who speak only one language. Language learning leads to more neural connections, more neural stability and more resilience to neural damage. Furthermore, research suggests that this bilingual effect is independent of your education, sex, occupation, or whether you live in an urban or rural setting. It was also found that there was no advantage in speaking more than two languages. Interestingly, the bilingual effect was evident both in those who were well educated and could speak two languages and in those who were illiterate and could speak two languages, suggesting that education alone can't explain the difference.[214]

However, the researchers queried whether people who can speak two languages have a different baseline cognitive ability – that is, do they start off with an advantage? They tested the cognitive abilities of a group of 853 children at the age of 11 and then retested them more than 60 years later. They found that those who were bilingual performed significantly better than would have been predicted from their baseline scores with the strongest effects on intelligence and reading. This positive effect was there even when they learned that second language in adulthood rather than as children.[215]

It is as if learning another language gives you 'a cognitive reserve' that helps to protect you against the changes that can occur during ageing.[216] Overall, the findings on language learning begs the question, could learning any other new skill give this same kind of benefit?

Using music

Research suggests that playing a musical instrument music when you are older can give you a 36 per cent lowered risk of developing dementia and cognitive impairment.[217] And even if you can't play an instrument, singing can help you to remember words more easily. Think how easily you can remember the words of songs that you sang years ago – and yet how much harder it often is to remember a poem or piece of prose that isn't set to music. Word sequences are far more memorable when they are sung rather than spoken.[218]

Everyday exercises

There's little doubt that the more you use your brain, the more you'll strengthen your cognitive reserve or brainpower against the symptoms of memory loss. Try a range of techniques to keep your brain alert. They don't have to be paper-based cognitive tasks: walking in a new park or taking up line dancing fire up new neural pathways that keep your brain in touch. Needing to remember the steps in a dance is also a wonderful workout for your brain – learning the flow and rhythm of the music stimulates cognitive activity, while learning and performing the steps is great for both your memory and your physical fitness. Active learning is the perfect complement for doing jigsaws, Sudoku and crosswords. Also try setting yourself little mental challenges: counting backwards from 100 in 2s, 3s or 4s is a good one, and you can make it harder by doing something else at the same time, such as tapping your foot. Or try the 'tip-of-the-tongue' game – think of a theme, such as 'food', and name as many items relevant to the theme as you can in one minute. Most people can do 30. Try to double it!

Chapter 13

Step 7: Testing, testing…

I'd like to start this chapter with a serious and quite philosophical question… Bearing in mind that studies show that Alzheimer's is now the most feared disease among the over-45s, and that you are indeed more likely to develop it if someone in your family has had it, would you really want your fears confirmed years before the condition becomes apparent and starts to affect your life?

A predictive test – telling you whether or not you are destined to develop dementia – is possible only for inherited Alzheimer's disease (which involves very rare mutations in three genes), and frontotemporal dementia (which involves mutations in at least six genes). There is – so far – no predictive test for the most common form of Alzheimer's disease, affecting about 520,000 people in the UK and usually starting over the age of 65. Because of this, at the time of writing, the NHS in the UK does not offer genetic testing for Alzheimer's disease, although it is possible to have the test (see p.45) through private clinics, including my own.

If you are considering having genetic testing, think first about the possible outcomes and the effects that each will have on you. Remember that you may get a result that indicates that you are susceptible to the disease, but that in no way guarantees that you will get it. On the one hand, the result then is inconclusive but, on the other, it is worrying. If you choose to disclose the fact that you have an increased risk, you might find that your employer begins to discriminate against you; or you might have trouble getting life or travel insurance, or even keeping hold of your driving license. There is a moratorium on the use of genetic information by UK insurance companies that remains in place until November 2019. The Alzheimer's Society is campaigning for this protection to continue – however, there is no guarantee that it will.

Blood tests to detect Alzheimer's

Having said all that, it is human nature for many people to want to know their risk and there are now several companies working towards finding blood tests that will detect Alzheimer's far sooner than (perhaps even years before) it would be possible to diagnose the condition through its symptoms. With early diagnosis comes the opportunity for early treatment.

One test, which aims to detect the disease up to ten years before a clinical diagnosis,[219] measures blood levels of a pathogenic protein called p-tau. Another, also aiming for a decade earlier for diagnosis, measures brain insulin resistance.[220] Yet another aims to identify Alzheimer's up to three years earlier by measuring the subject's levels of blood fats.[221]

All of these tests are still at the stages of being replicated and validated, so none of them are yet available except under research conditions, but in several years' time we may see some, or all, in hospitals and clinics.

Testing for heavy metals

We know that there is a connection between toxicity from heavy metals and your risk of developing Alzheimer's (see p.142), so it makes sense that analysing how toxic you are can provide an indicator of risk. The easiest and most sensitive way to test is through hair analysis, which can accurately measure your body's levels of aluminium, mercury, lead, arsenic, cadmium and nickel.

There is also a urine test for heavy metals but it doesn't measure the organic form of mercury, methylmercury, which is found in fish; and urine is not the normal route for mercury excretion, so you would not get a true reading. There is also a lack of agreement on the significance of blood levels of mercury.

Furthermore, hair analysis doesn't require any trip to a clinic or lab – you just collect your hair sample yourself, send it off and wait for the test results to come back to you. (See Resources page 172.)

Testing for nutrient deficiencies and imbalances

At my clinic we do blood tests for all the important vitamins, minerals and essential fats (i.e. calcium, chromium, copper, zinc, iron, magnesium (red cell), selenium, manganese, vitamins A, E and D, omega 3 and omega 6) to make sure you are not deficient in any of them. We can then tailor a nutritional programme (looking at diet and supplements) according to your individual needs, as well as general health.

Testing for copper and zinc

In order to be in good health you need good levels of certain minerals, particularly those that assist in the smooth functioning of the nervous system and that provide antioxidant protection against free radicals. A ratio of copper to zinc that is higher than 1:3 is cause for concern in terms of your risk of developing Alzheimer's (and I would encourage you to take zinc supplements to improve the ratio, raising zinc and lowering copper). You can test for mineral levels either through a hair analysis or (and I believe more accurately) through a blood test.

Testing is useful as part of the process to find out where you stand now, put a dietary and supplement programme in place to correct any deficiencies or imbalances, and then do a retest to make sure that your nutritional programme has corrected those deficiencies or imbalances. The aim after that is to maintain those levels within the normal range, perhaps lowering the amounts of some supplements to sustain their levels rather than continuing to increase them.

Omega 3 and 6 test

Of the all the tests that I would recommend for brain health, the omega 3 and 6 test has to be the most important. Your levels of omega 3, particularly DHA, are crucial for blood flow in your brain (and also your heart). Omega 3 also helps prevent and reduce the build-up of beta-amyloid plaques, and acts as an anti-inflammatory. A test for omega 6 looks for levels that are too high, which can cause inflammation and abnormal blood clotting.

You can come to my clinic to test your blood levels of omega 3 and omega 6 and there is also a simple finger-prick blood test for fatty acids that you can send away for and then do at home. The test is called Omega 3 Deficiency Test (you can order it online; see Resources page 172). It will give you your blood levels of:

- Omega 3 and omega 6 as a ratio of one to the other
- DHA
- EPA
- Trans fats
- Omega 9
- Alpha linolenic acid (ALA)
- Saturated fats

You are then sent a report that will include dietary and supplement recommendations to correct any deficiencies or imbalances.

Vitamin D

Deficiencies in vitamin D are linked to many health issues, including your brain function (see p.114) – but you also need to make sure your level is not too high. Supplementation is all well and good – as long as you're mindful of your levels so that you stop taking supplements if too much vitamin D begins to circulate in your system. This means having a simple blood test, as part of your overall nutritional analysis, or doing a home finger-prick test (see p.172)

Vitamin D is a fat-soluble vitamin, so results from tests in my own clinic that show some people who supplement the vitamin, but remain deficient in it are particularly interesting. This could signal that a person is not absorbing fats efficiently, in which case I would recommend a digestive stool test (see over page).

The importance of nutritional testing

I think the benefits of nutritional testing are huge. Over the last 30 years, increased types of nutritional tests have changed how we individualise a person's diet and supplement recommendations according to their specific deficiencies and imbalances.

Years ago, it was fashionable for people to be on an anti-*candida* diet, for example, just because they 'felt' they had the symptoms or because they ticked boxes on a *Candida* questionnaire. This is not scientific. I think it is important for an independent and accredited laboratory to test samples (blood, urine, hair, stool or saliva) to check for nutritional deficiencies or toxicity and then to report back the findings.

As a result of all the scientific developments, we now have many tools to assess your health. But, before you embark on a series of nutritional testing, if you feel unwell or concerned about your health in any way, start with your doctor. Tests from your doctor will be designed to rule out anything immediately serious. If you are then told that everything is 'normal', that is when I think you need to look at your health from another angle – looking at deficiencies, the efficiency of your digestive system, whether you are stressed, your level of heavy metals and more if needed. See Resources pages 172-173 for information on how to test your nutritional wellbeing.

Testing for homocysteine levels

A homocysteine level over 14 mmol/L can double your risk of developing Alzheimer's (see p.107).[222] At my clinic, we test for homocysteine levels at the same time as testing for nutrient deficiencies and imbalances, but, as with the omega 3 test, there is also a simple home finger-prick test you can do. (See Resources page 172 for more information).

Testing for blood sugar and insulin resistance

In Chapter 4 we learned that some people now refer to Alzheimer's as type 3 diabetes, marking just how important it is to understand the nature of your blood sugar and insulin resistance in order to assess risk of developing the disease. The test most clinics will use to assess your blood glucose levels is called the HbA1c (glycosylated haemoglobin). Rather than looking at fasting blood glucose levels, the HbA1c assesses the amount of glucose attached to part of your red blood cells to give an indicator of your blood glucose levels over the past two or three months. An HbA1c level of 48 mmol/mol (6.5 per cent) or more is considered a diagnosis of diabetes.

If the HbA1c level is 42–47 mmol/mol (6–6.4 per cent), you'll receive a diagnosis of pre-diabetes.

For a more comprehensive test, which measures HbA1c plus insulin, cholesterol (and your ratios of good to bad cholesterol), plus highly sensitive C-reactive protein (a marker of inflammation), you would have a fasting blood test. This comes in the form of a kit that you take first thing in the morning, before you eat or drink anything, to your local practice nurse or doctor. At the surgery you give a small quantity of blood that is sent to a laboratory for analysis. The results are sent back to you with explanation of what they mean. For more information on this test, see Resources page 172.

Digestive stool analysis

Beneficial bacteria (probiotics), which live naturally in your digestive system, have an anti-inflammatory effect on your body. This is important for both your brain health and your immune system. Probiotics help to manufacture the B vitamins that are important in controlling levels of toxic homocysteine in your body, and they help your body in its work to detoxify your system, encouraging it to eliminate heavy metals, and in particular mercury.[223]

Your results not only include your levels of beneficial bacteria, such as *lactobacillus* and *bifidobacteria* but also levels of 'negative' pathogenic bacteria and yeasts like *candida*. The lab also checks for parasites and this is important if you have had a previous case of food poisoning and feel that your digestive function is not as it should be as you may still have a 'bug' in there. The test also shows whether you can digest and absorb your food efficiently across fats, carbohydrates and protein.

This test is also useful if you have IBS or any digestive problems like bloating, flatulence and especially if you have had a colonoscopy and told everything is fine. A colonoscopy is important to rule out any serious problems but it is looking more at the structure of your digestive system, are there any polyps for example? The digestive stool test is looking at your digestive function. This stool test is also important if you struggle to gain weight even though you are eating well, as you may have a problem with malabsorption.

The test involves collecting three stool samples, according to instructions that come with the testing kit (see Resources page 172 for how to get one of these), at home and sending them off – it's important to have three samples in order to ensure accurate results.

Any problems that are identified can be helped with dietary and supplement recommendations and then you would have a re-test a few months later to make sure that all the levels are back to normal.

Antibiotics and good bacteria

Antibiotic medicine wipes out good bacteria in your gut, so if you're on medication for any reason, even if it seems unrelated to your brain health, it's important to have a digestive stool analysis if you're worried about Alzheimer's or dementia.

Gluten test

The relationship between coeliac disease and cognitive decline is still under investigation, but some research suggests that those who have coeliac disease (a digestive disorder characterised by an intolerance to gluten) may be at greater risk of developing Alzheimer's or other forms of dementia. For this reason, knowing whether or not you have coeliac disease can provide a marker for your likelihood to suffer cognitive decline.

The gluten test is a simple blood test that looks at tissue transglutaminase and endomysial antibodies. Having a positive result overall gives an accuracy of 99 per cent that you have coeliac disease, although occasionally (rarely nowadays) you may have to have a small intestine biopsy to confirm the diagnosis. If you think you might have coeliac disease you need to be tested before you start to eliminate gluten from your diet, otherwise the test can give a false negative reading because your gluten-free diet will stop your body producing the antibodies that are picked up by the blood test.

You can also have non-coeliac gluten sensitivity without having full-blown coeliac disease. So you might have symptoms that are similar to those experienced in coeliac disease, but a blood test will be negative for antibodies and you won't have damage to the small intestine. It is thought that gluten sensitivity can affect up to 10 per cent of people compared to just 1 per cent for coeliac disease.

The blood test I use in my clinic can differentiate between having coeliac and being gluten sensitive, depending on which markers are positive and which are negative (see Resources page 172).

Adrenal stress test including melatonin

We talked about how important it is to control stress in Chapter 10 and there is a simple laboratory test that measures cortisol and melatonin and it uses samples of saliva.

Although adrenaline is also a stress hormone it is so short lived that it makes it almost impossible to test. Using saliva samples instead of blood means that a number of samples can be collected over the course of the day to look at what is going on with the circadian rhythm of these hormones. If you would like to organise this test then please go to the Resources page 172.

Genetic testing for general wellbeing

In the last chapter we talked about APOE testing, specifically looking at markers that can predict Alzheimer's, but there are other genetic tests that I also think are helpful. There are some genes, that can be measured, that can give you practical information about how you can make simple changes to your diet and lifestyle that can change your present and future health. Anything that keeps you generally well, keeps all your cells, including those in your nervous system and brain, functioning efficiently for as long as possible.

The genetic test I use in my clinic gives you guidance on what you should eat and how you should exercise, according to your genetic make-up. It measures 45 genetic markers that tell you:

- Whether you have a greater need for certain nutrients such as omega 3, vitamin D and B vitamin levels.

- How well you detoxify.

- Your sensitivity to caffeine and salt.

- Whether you are at risk of being lactose intolerant.

- Your sensitivity to saturated fat.

- Whether you are at risk of having coeliac disease.

- Your ideal way to eat – for example, low fat or high protein.

- Your antioxidants needs.

- What type of exercise (cardiovascular or weight training) suits your genetic make-up.

Knowing this information is important for your general health because you may need higher levels of certain nutrients, or you may need to be careful about gluten or dairy or your body might need extra help detoxifying.

It is also important for your future health because what you learn about your genetic make-up can help you work on prevention.

Research has also shown that information about your genes can be particularly helpful if you have failed in all your weight loss attempts so far. Results have shown that if people follow a diet based on their genetic results then they lose 33 per cent more weight than those who are on an untailored diet.[224]

If you intend to have a genetic test, it's important that you have professional advice when interpreting the results (see Resources page 172).

Brain Protection Profile

To make the process much easier, my clinic uses an exclusive Brain Protection Profile which includes the four most important tests for brain health.

- Hair analysis to check for heavy metals including mercury, aluminium, cadmium, lead, arsenic and nickel.

- Testing for nutrient deficiencies – this blood test checks for deficiencies and imbalances; in calcium, chromium, copper, zinc, iron, magnesium (red cell), selenium, manganese, vitamins A, E and D, omega 3 and omega 6; to make sure you are not deficient in any of them.

- Homocysteine – to make sure this amino acid is not too high.

- HbA1c – to check for your average blood glucose levels over the last three months.

We start by sending you the kit to collect the hair sample and also organise the blood test to be taken either in London or local to you, a questionnaire is also sent out to you to complete before the consultation. On it, you are asked to list any health concerns, and give details of your typical diet and lifestyle habits, including how much stress you are under. We analyse the answers before you come in to see us, so that we understand what further questions we need to ask to ensure you get the best from your consultation.

During the consultation, your results are discussed and you will be given copies of those results to keep. You will be given advice on what to eat and what to avoid in order to improve your health now and for the future. Information will also be given as to how to correct any deficiencies or imbalances that have come up from the test results. If you are interested in having the Brain Protection Profile then contact my clinic directly see Resources page 172.

How to organise a test

All of the tests mentioned in this chapter are available at my clinic (see Resources page 172 for contact details), and the online postal laboratory tests are available at www.naturalhealthpractice.com. Consultations via Skype or telephone make nutritional advice available to you wherever you are, but if you would prefer to visit, face-to-face consultations are available in the clinic, too.

If you want to know if my clinic can help you then you are always welcome to phone just to talk things through before making a decision (see Resources page 172 for contact details). Also a consultation can be helpful as I realise the list of tests is quite extensive and in a consultation we can work out more specifically what you may need.

Conclusion

And finally…

I think what has become obvious from the information and research in this book is that dementia and Alzheimer's are multi-factorial. There is no magic bullet or single drug to treat memory loss. Instead, you need to put into place a strategy that combines diet, supplements, exercise, brain training and lifestyle changes that we know can improve brain function.

From a medical perspective, understanding and treating Alzheimer's or dementia is really difficult, because drug companies are looking for a single miracle cure and research tends to want to compare a single treatment versus a single placebo – which is hard to do with a multi-factorial illness. Nonetheless, whatever approach researchers are taking, nothing stops you taking all the self-help steps available to you to try to reduce your risk.

Treating dementia requires a personalised approach. By targeting all the different aspects that relate to you at the same time, you have the best chance of making positive improvements to your condition, slowing its onset, or even perhaps preventing it altogether. Remember, do what suits you – perhaps your vitamin D levels are fine (no need to supplement), whereas for someone else they are not; perhaps you are intolerant to gluten (you need to avoid it), whereas someone else may be able to eat it without any ill effects. Consider your body, your lifestyle and your personal wellbeing and tailor your approach to protect your cognitive function in a way that is personal to you.

Starting on a path to individualised wellbeing produces a domino effect throughout your mind and body. As you start to eat well, you gain more energy and then realise you can do a bit more exercise, which lifts your mood and then you are able to cope more with stress, so you eat fewer sugary or otherwise unhealthy comfort foods – which means you then have more energy and so on... I see this wonderful effect in my clinic every day.

A large-scale human trial – on 1,300 people aged 60 to 77 – undertaken in Finland in 2015, studied the effects of a combination of regular exercise, good diet, brain training and social activities over the course of two years. The researchers found that if you make changes in several risk factors all at the same time (even if they are small changes), there is a protective effect on brain function.[225] Those at risk of dementia who were put on this two-year lifestyle programme performed 25 per cent better overall on brain tests than those given basic health advice. They were also 83 per cent better at organising their thoughts and a whopping 150 per cent better at processing information.

A more individualised programme of diet and lifestyle changes has been tried out in the USA on a small number of people (only ten) with excellent results.[226] The ten participants had memory problems that were so significant they had to give up work. After following the diet and lifestyle programme given to them, every one of them managed to reverse their memory loss and cognitive impairment so that they could return to work. Interestingly, nine of the ten people carried the APOE4 gene, with five of them having the two copies that put them at a much higher risk (10 to 12 fold) of developing Alzheimer's. Significantly, the study found that you have to sustain any diet and lifestyle changes that reverse cognitive impairment for life. One of the participants stopped their programme after three months, leading to a rapid relapse in memory function.

Following my 7-step brain protection plan has enormous benefits not only for your brain health, but also for your general health. These same steps can protect you from other degenerative illnesses, such as type 2 diabetes, heart disease and cancer. You have nothing to lose and everything to gain.

Be realistic. Making lifestyle changes may require a bit of effort at first but you will notice fairly quickly improvements in your energy, skin, mood, digestion and myriad other physical effects that might have seemed unconnected. Rest assured that, behind the scenes, your brain will also be reaping the rewards of the work you have put in – you will probably notice quickly that you feel more alert and focused.

Get started!

You can protect your brain at any time – no matter what age you are, it is never too late to prioritise your brain health. While research into Alzheimer's and dementia is ongoing, and we're making new discoveries all the time, one thing we already know for sure is that positive, brain-healthy changes to diet and lifestyle do make a difference – not only in terms of how you feel your brain is working (your clarity of thought, your concentration and your memory), but also in terms of what a doctor can actually see on a brain scan.[227]

So, in summary, here are the 7 steps that I think are the most important steps you need to follow in order to protect your brain.

Step 1: Change your diet

This is most important part of my brain protection plan. What you eat is the foundation of your health both physically and mentally. The quality of what you eat and drink is powerful medicine and has a profound effect on the different biochemical processes not only in your body but also in your mind. Choose the best-quality food you can and choose organic foods where possible. Avoid added chemicals in your food and drink – artificial sweeteners, colourings, preservatives and additives are all off the menu. Then, follow these and the other steps outlined in Chapter 6;

- Eat unrefined carbohydrates – reduce or eliminate white bread, pasta and rice.
- Avoid food and drink with added sugar.
- Eat more healthy omega 3 fats, including more oily fish.
- Include good amounts of fruits and vegetables.
- Cut back on unhealthy fats, such as trans fats.
- Cut down on, or eliminate, caffeine.

- Reduce or eliminate gluten – you might need to eliminate it completely depending on testing.

- Reduce or eliminate alcohol.

- Leave 12 hours without eating overnight and don't eat in the three hours running up to bedtime.

Step 2: Supplement your nutrition

What you will need in the way of extra nutrients will depend on whether you have been checked for any deficiencies and need more of certain vitamins or minerals for a few months in order to correct low nutrient levels. What you need will also depend on the reason that you are following my brain protection plan. You are going to need a more intensive programme of supplements if you have already been diagnosed with early stage Alzheimer's or dementia compared to someone who is working on prevention. A good supplement programme would comprise a multivitamin and mineral designed for brain health (such as NHP's Advanced Brain and Memory Support; see P.172) and additional omega 3, vitamin C and probiotics.

Step 3: Exercise

Exercise (along with your healthy diet) helps to keep your weight at optimal levels and helps to control your blood sugar. We know from Chapter 9 that exercise not only helps with your memory, but also increases the size of the hippocampus, so it is causing definite and very positive physical changes in your brain. Make it part of your daily routine. Find an exercise that you enjoy, because that way you are more likely to keep doing it.

Step 4: Manage your stress (and your sleep)

We know that stress can increase your risk of Alzheimer's, so stress management is a crucial part of your plan. Use meditation or yoga to help control stress.Make sure you have eliminated caffeine and all other stimulants (including alcohol and cigarettes), as stimulants make you feel more stressed. Balancing your blood sugar (the dietary changes will do this) will also regulate your stress hormones.

Good amounts of good-quality sleep are important for helping to clear away beta-amyloid plaques from your brain. Being less stressed helps you sleep better, as it stops you being 'tired but wired'.

Step 5: Clean your environment

Reduce your toxic load – and protect the health of your liver – by ensuring that you avoid pesticides and other pollutants as often and as much as you can. This includes reducing the amount of alcohol you consume (or giving it up altogether if you can) and definitely stopping smoking.

Step 6: Train your brain

As well as keeping your body active, you need to keep your brain active, too. Choose brain activities that you enjoy and that way you are more likely to continue them. You could try brain-training apps (a lot of them are free until you reach certain levels), learning a new instrument or language, or a new skill of any kind.

Step 7: Embrace testing

In more than 30 years in clinical practice I have to say that being able to test for different nutritional factors has made such a difference, because it enables me to personalise nutrition. I am able to tailor not only a patient's diet, but also a supplement programme so that my patients are taking exactly what they need, according to each individual's test results.

If you intend to test only a couple of things, I would suggest the most important ones are your levels of omega 3 and 6, vitamin D and homocysteine. A simple home finger-prick blood test is suitable for all three, so you can organise to have the tests by post if you prefer (see p.172). However, if you want a more personalised approach, it is better to have the Brain Protection Profile which includes a consultation (with a Skype or phone appointment if you can't come in person) so that we can focus on your specific, individual needs.

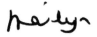

Resources

Glenville Nutrition Clinics
Natural Healthcare For Women

Consultations:

If you would like to have a consultation (either in person, on the telephone or by Skype), then please feel free to phone my clinic for an appointment.

All the qualified nutritionists who work in my UK and Irish clinics have been trained by me in my specific approach to nutrition.

The clinics are located in:

UK - Harley Street, London and Tunbridge Wells, Kent.

To book a personal or telephone appointment at any of these clinics, or for more information, please contact us at:

Glenville Nutrition Clinic　　**Tel:** 01892 515905

14 St John's Road,　　　　　　　**Int. Tel:** +44 1 892 515905

Tunbridge Wells,　　　　　　　　**Email:** health@marilynglenville.com

Kent, TN4 9NP.　　　　　　　　　**Website:** www.marilynglenville.com

Ireland - Dublin, Galway, Kilkenny and Cork

To book a personal or telephone appointment at any of these clinics, or for more information, please contact us at:

Website: www.glenvillenutrition.ie
Tel: 01 402 0777 | **Int. Tel:** + 353 1 402 0777

Supplements and Tests: The Natural Health Practice (NHP) is my supplier of choice for all the supplements and tests by post mentioned in this book. They only carry products that I use in my clinics and are in the correct form and use the highest quality ingredients. For more information, please contact:

Website: www.naturalhealthpractice.com
Tel: 01892 507598 | **Int. Tel:** + 44 1 892 507598

Workshops and Talks: I frequently give workshops and talks. See my website for my upcoming schedule: www.marilynglenville.com. If you would like to organise a workshop/talk near you, I would be happy to come and speak - call my clinic and ask for information about how to arrange this.

If you have enjoyed this book then please send a review.

I also invite you to join me on Facebook and Twitter for more information, tips and updates on my work.

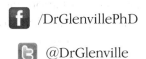 /DrGlenvillePhD

@DrGlenville

Free Health Tips

If you would like to receive my exclusive Health Tips by email, drop me a line at health@marilynglenville.com. Just mention "Free Health Tips" in the subject line and you will be added to my special list to receive regular health tips and other useful information.

Other Books By Dr Marilyn Glenville PhD

Fat around the Middle – how to lose that bulge for good

Natural Alternatives to Sugar

Getting Pregnant Faster

Natural Solutions to the Menopause

Healthy Eating for the Menopause Cookbook

Natural Solutions to PCOS

Natural Solutions to IBS

The Natural Health Bible for Women

Osteoporosis – how to prevent, treat and reverse it

The Nutritional Health Handbook for Women

Overcoming PMS The Natural Way

Natural Alternatives to HRT

Natural Solutions to Infertility

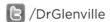 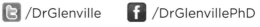

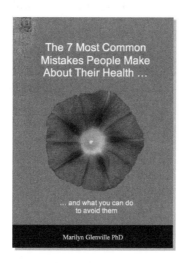

Other books by Dr Marilyn Glenville PhD

THE NATURAL HEALTH BIBLE FOR WOMEN

A practical, easy-to-use reference book guiding you step-by-step through the unique aspects of a woman's body. You will learn how nutrition, lifestyle and natural therapies can maximise your health and vitality

FAT AROUND THE MIDDLE

A practical action plan showing how you can get rid of that bulge once and for all.... and it's not just about diet!

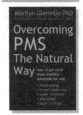

OVERCOMING PMS THE NATURAL WAY

Are you one of the 70% to 90% of women who suffer every month with premenstrual symptoms?... At last a groundbreaking approach to eliminating these symptoms for good.

GETTING PREGNANT FASTER

Boost your fertility in just 3 months and discover the "8 steps to fertility" plan that will help you to get pregnant faster.

NATURAL SOLUTIONS TO PCOS

Beat PCOS and enjoy a symptom-free life, naturally. Dr Marilyn Glenville PhD has helped thousands of women overcome PCOS and now you too can benefit from her unique, nutritional programme.

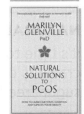

NUTRITIONAL HEALTH HANDBOOK FOR WOMEN

Everything you need to know on the most effective ways to treat all aspects of women's health - naturally.

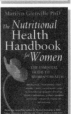

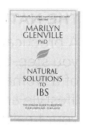
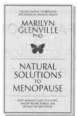
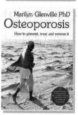
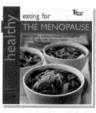
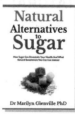

References

Chapter 2

Page 26 1 Hye A et al, 2014, Plasma proteins predict conversion to dementia from prodromal disease. *Alzheimers Dement*, 10, 6, 799-807

Page 27 2 Presented at the Alzheimer's Association International Conference in Toronto July 2016

3 Gupta V et al, 2016, One protein, multiple pathologies: multifaceted involvement of amyloid β in neurodegenerative disorders of the brain and retina, *Curr Alzheimer Res*, Jun 2 (Epub ahead of print)

4 Frost S et al, 2016, Alzheimer's disease and the early signs of age-related macular degeneration, *Curr Alzheimer Res*, Jun 2 (Epub ahead of print).

Page 28 5 Velayudhan L et al, 2015, Pattern of Smell Identification Impairment in Alzheimer's Disease, *J Alzheimer's Dis*, 46, 2, 381-7

6 Brooke, P, Bullock R, 1999, Validation of The 6 Item Cognitive Impairment Test. *Int J Geriatr Psychiatry*, 14, 936-940

Chapter 3

Page 34 7 Vom Berg J et al, 2012, Inhibition of IL-12/IL-23 signaling reduces Alzheimer's disease-like pathology and cognitive decline, *Nat Med*, 18, 12, 1812-9

8 Olmos-Alonso A et al, 2016, Pharmacological targeting of CSF1R inhibits microglial proliferation and prevents the progression of Alzheimer's-like pathology, *Brain*, 139, Pt3, 891-907

9 Yan Z and Baolu Z, 2013, Review Article, Oxidative Stress and the Pathogenesis of Alzheimer's Disease. *Oxidative Medicine and Cellular Longevity*, Article ID 316523

Page 35 10 Bayer-Carter JL et al, 2011, Diet intervention and cerebrospinal fluid biomarkers in amnestic mild cognitive impairment. *Arch Neurol*, 68, 6, 743-52

Page 35   11 Talbot, K et al, 2012, Demonstrated brain insulin resistance in Alzheimer's disease patients is associated with IGF-1 resistance, IRS-1 dysregulation, and cognitive decline. *J Clin Invest*, 122, 1316-1338)

Page 37   12 Kumar DK et al, 2016, Amyloid-β peptide protects against microbial infection in mouse and worm models of Alzheimer's disease, *Sci Transl Med*, 8, 340,

13 Viiaya Kumar DK et al, 2016, Alzheimer's disease: the potential therapeutic role of the natural antibiotic amyloid-β peptide, *Neurodegener Dis Manag*, September 7, (Epub ahead of print)

Page 38   14 Soscia SJ et al, 2010, The Alzheimer's disease-associated amyloid beta-protein is an antimicrobial peptide. *PLoS One*, 5, 3, e9505

15 Pisa D, 2015, Different Brain Regions are Infected with Fungi in Alzheimer's disease, *Scientific Reports*, 5, 15015

Chapter 4

Page 40   16 http://www.world-heart-federation.org/cardiovascular-health/cardiovascular-disease-risk-factors/

17 Laws KR et al, 2016, Sex differences in cognitive impairment in Alzheimer's disease, *World J Psychiatry*, 6, 1, 54-65

Page 41   18 Findings presented at the Alzheimer's Association International Conference in Toronto July 2016

19 Greendale GA et al, 2009, Effects of the menopause transition and hormone use on cognitive performance in midlife women, *Neurology*, 72, 21, 1850-7

Page 42   20 Mielke MM et al, 2014, Clinical epidemiology of Alzheimer's disease: assessing sex and gender differences, *Clin Epidemiol*, 6, 37-48

Page 44   21 http://www.ashg.org/pdf/cdc%20gene-environment%20interaction%20fact%20sheet.pdf

Page 48   22 Macauley SL et al, 2015, Hyperglycemia modulates extracellular amyloid beta concentrations and neuronal activity *in vivo*, *J Clin Invest*, 125, 6, 2463-7

Chapter 4

Page 48   23 Lin F, American Association for the Advancement of Science conference Feb 2016 Bernabei R et al, 2014, Hearing loss and cognitive decline in older adults: questions and answers. *Aging Clin Exp Res*, 26, 6, 567-73

Page 49   24 Gallacher J et al, 2012, Auditory threshold, phonologic demand, and incident dementia. *Neurology*. 79, 15, 1583-90

         25 Ide M et al, 2016, Periodontitis and Cognitive Decline in Alzheimer's Disease, *PLoS One*, 11, 3.

Page 50   26 Gomm W et al, 2016, Association of Proton Pump Inhibitors With Risk of Dementia: A Pharmacoepidemiological Claims Data Analysis, *JAMA Neurol*, 73, 4, 410-6

         27 Badiola N et al, 2013, The proton-pump inhibitor lansoprazole enhances amyloid beta production, *PLos One*, 8, 3, e58837

         28 Farrella CP et al, 2011, Proton Pump Inhibitors Interfere With Zinc Absorption and Zinc Body Stores, *Gastroenterology Research*, 2011;4(6):243-251

Page 51   29 Risacher SL et al, 2016, Association Between Anticholinergic Medication Use and Cognition, Brain Metabolism, and Brain Atrophy in Cognitively Normal Older Adults, *JAMA Neurol*, 73, 6 721-32

         30 Nouchi R et al, 2014, Four weeks of combination exercise training improved executive functions, episodic memory, and processing speed in healthy elderly people: evidence from a randomized controlled trial, *Age*, 36, 2, 787-99

Page 53   31 Gaiewski PD et al, 2014, Toxoplasma gondii impairs memory in infected seniors, *Brain Behav Immun*, 36, 193-9

         32 Gaiewski PD et al, 2014, Toxoplasma gondii impairs memory in infected seniors, *Brain Behav Immun*, 36, 193-9

         33 Mendy A et al, 2015, Immediate rather than delayed memory impairment in older adults with latent toxoplasmosis, *Brain Behav Immun*, 45, 36-40

Chapter 5

Page 56   34 Fu AK et al, 2016, IL-33 ameliorates Alzheimer's disease-like pathology and cognitive decline, *Proc Natl Acad Sci*, 113,19: E2705-13

Page 56   35 Heppner F et al, 2015, Immune attack: the role of
inflammation in Alzheimer disease, *Nature Reviews
Neuroscience*,16,358-372

Page 57   36 Atri A et al, 2015, Cumulative, additive benefits of memantine-
donepezil combination over component monotherapies in
moderate to severe Alzheimer's dementia: a pooled area
under the curve analysis, *Alzheimer's Research and Therapy*,
7. 28

Page 58   37 Ye F et al, 2016, Impact of Insulin Sensitizers on the Incidence
of Dementia: A Meta-Analysis, *Dement Geriatr Cogn Disord*,
41, 5-6, 251-60

          38 Minter MR et al, 2016, These findings suggest the gut
microbiota community diversity can regulate host innate
immunity mechanisms that impact Aβ amyloidosis, *Sci Rep*,
July 21, 6, 30028

Page 59   39 Sevigny J et al, 2016, The antibody aducanumab reduces Aβ
plaques in Alzheimer's disease. *Nature*, 537, 7618, 50-6

          40 Piazza F and Winblad B, 2016, Amyloid-Related Imaging
Abnormalities (ARIA) in Immunotherapy Trials for Alzheimer's
Disease: Need for Prognostic Biomarkers? *J Alzheimer's Dis*, 52, 2,
417-20

          41 Godyn J et al, 2016, Therapeutic strategies for Alzheimer's
disease in clinical trials, *Pharmacol Rep*, 68, 1, 127-38

          42 Fu AK et al, 2016, IL-33 ameliorates Alzheimer's disease-like
pathology and cognitive decline, *Proc Natl Acad Sci USA*, 113,
19, E2705-13

Page 60   43 Gauthier S, presented at the Alzheimer's Association
International Conference in Toronto July 2016 and Wischik
CM et al, 2015, Tau aggregation inhibitor therapy: an
exploratory phase 2 study in mild or moderate Alzheimer's
disease. *J Alzheimers Dis*, 44, 2, 705-20

Chapter 6

Page 63   44 Scarmeas N et al, 2009, Mediterranean diet and mild cognitive
impairment. *Archives of Neurology*. 66 (2), 216-25.

Page 64   45 Morris MC et al, 2015, MIND diet associated with reduced
incidence of Alzheimer's disease, *Alzheimer's Dement*, 11, 9,
1997-14

Chapter 6

Page 65   46 Bredesen DE, 2014, Reversal of cognitive decline: a novel therapeutic program. *Aging (Albany NY)*, 6, 9, 707-17

          47 Brewer GJ, 2015, Copper-2 Ingestion, Plus Increased Meat Eating Leading to Increased Copper Absorption, Are Major Factors Behind the Current Epidemic of Alzheimer's Disease. *Nutrients*, 7(12):10053-64

Page 66   48 Poly C et al, 2011, The relation of dietary choline to cognitive performance and white-matter hyperintensity in the Framingham Offspring Cohort, *Am J Clin Nutr*, 94, 6, 1584-91

          49 Fernandez ML, 2012, Effects of eggs on plasma lipoproteins in healthy populations, *Food Funct*, 1, 2, 156-60

          50 Chandalia M et al, 2000, Beneficial effects of high dietary fiber intake in patients with type 2 diabetes mellitus, *NEJM*, 342, 1392-8

Page 67   51 Jayagopal V et al, 2002, Beneficial effects of soy phytoestrogen intake in postmenopausal women with type 2 diabetes, *Diabetes Care*, 25, 1709-14

Page 69   52 Bazzano LA et al, 2008, Intake of fruit, vegetables and fruit juices and risk of diabetes in women, *Diabetes Care*, 31, 7, 1311-7

Page 70   53 Welsh JA et al, 2010, Caloric sweetener consumption and dyslipidemia among US adults, *JAMA*, 303, 15, 1490-7

          54 Crane PK et al, 2013, Glucose levels and risk of dementia, *Eng J Med*, 369, 6, 540-8

Page 71   55 Hill S et al, 2014, The effect of non-caloric sweeteners on cognition, choice and post-consumption satisfaction, *Appetite*, 83, 82-88

          56 Lee SJ et al, 2009, Cell Press, Spoonful Of Sugar' Makes The Worms' Life Span Go Down, *Science Daily*, November 5

          57 West RK et al, 2014, Dietary advanced glycation end products are associated with decline in memory in young elderly, *Mech Ageing Dev*, 140, 10-2

          58 Beilharz JE et al, 2016, Short-term exposure to a diet high in fat and sugar, or liquid sugar, selectively impairs hippocampal-dependent memory, with differential impacts on inflammation, *Behav Brain Res*, 306, 1-7

Page 72   59 West RK et al, 2014, Dietary advanced glycation end products
           are associated with decline in memory in young elderly, *Mech
           Ageing Dev*, 140, 10-2

           60 Beilharz JE et al, 2016, Short-term exposure to a diet
           high in fat and sugar, or liquid sugar, selectively impairs
           hippocampal-dependent memory, with differential impacts
           on inflammation, *Behav Brain Res*, 306, 1-7

Page 73   61 Keast DR et al, 2010, Snacking is associated with reduced risk
           of overweight and reduced abdominal obesity in adolescents:
           National Health and Nutrition Examination Survey (NHANES)
           1999–2004, *Am J Clin Nutr*, 92, 4280435

Page 74   62 Bitel CL et al, 2012, Amyloid-β and tau pathology of Alzheimer's
           disease induced by diabetes in a rabbit animal model. *J Alzheimers
           Dis*, 32, 2, 291-305

           63 Talbot, K et al, 2012, Demonstrated brain insulin resistance
           in Alzheimer's disease patients is associated with IGF-1
           resistance, IRS-1 dysregulation, and cognitive decline. *J. Clin.
           Invest*. 122, 1316-1338

           64 Bayer-Carter JL et al, 2011, Diet intervention and
           cerebrospinal fluid biomarkers in amnestic mild cognitive
           impairment. *Arch Neurol*, 68, 6, 743-52

           65 APOE ε4 and the associations of seafood and long-chain
           omega 3 fatty acids with cognitive decline. Van de Rest O et al,
           2016, *Neurology,* 186, 22, 2063-70

Page 75   66 Yashodhara BM et al, 2009, Omega 3 fatty acids: a
           comprehensive review of their role in health and disease,
           Postgrad Med J, 85, 1000, 84-90

           67 Kiecolt-Glaser et al, 2007, Depressive symptoms, omega
           3:omega 6 fatty acids and inflammation in older adults,
           Psychom Med, 69, 3, 217-24

           68 Schaefer EJ et al, 2006, Plasma phosphatidylcholine
           docosahexaenoic acid content and risk of dementia and
           Alzheimer disease: the Framingham Heart Study. *Arch
           Neurol*, 63, 11, 1545-1550

Chapter 6

Page 75   69 Ma QL et al, 2007, Omega 3 fatty acid docosahexaenoic acid increases SorLA/LR11, a sorting protein with reduced expression in sporadic Alzheimer's disease (AD): relevance to AD prevention, *J Neurosci*, 27, 52, 14299-307

70 Simopoulos AP, 2011, Evolutionary aspects of diet: the omega 6/omega 3 ratio and the brain *Mol Neurobiol*, 44, 2, 203-15

Page 76   71 Gerster H, 1998, Can adults adequately convert alpha-linolenic acid (18:3n-3) to eicosapentaenoic acid (20:5n-3) and docosahexaenoic acid (22:6n-3)?, *Int J Vitam Nutr Res*, 68, 3, 159-73

Page 77   72 Cunnane SC et al, 2016, Can ketones compensate for deteriorating brain glucose uptake during aging? Implications for the risk and treatment of Alzheimer's disease, *Ann NY Acad Sci*, 1367, 1,12-20

73 Hu Yang I et al, 2015, Coconut oil: non-alternative drug treatment against Alzheimer's disease, *Nutr Hosp*, 32, 6, 2822-7

74 Cardoso DA et al, 2015, A coconut extra virgin oil-rich diet increases HDL cholesterol and decreases waist circumference and body mass in coronary artery disease patients, *Nutr Hosp*, 32, 5, 2144-52

Page 79   75 Kavanagh et al, 2007, Trans fat diet induces abdominal obesity and changes in insulin sensitivity in monkeys, *Obesity*, 15, 1675-1684

76 Whitmer RA et al, 2008. Central obesity and increased risk of dementia more than three decades later, *Neurology*, 71, 14, 1057-64

77 Salmeron J et al, 2001, Dietary fat intake and risk of type 2 diabetes in women, *Am J Clin Nutr*, 73, 6, 1019-26

78 Ginter E, Simko V, 2016, New data on harmful effects of trans-fatty acids, *Bratisl Lek Listy*. 2 117(5):251-3.

Page 80   79 Qin B et al, 2010, Cinnamon: potential role in the prevention of insulin resistance, metabolic syndrome and type 2 diabetes, *J Diabetes Sci Technol*, 4, 3, 685-93

Page 80   80 Madhavadas S, Subramanian S, 2016, Cognition enhancing effect of the aqueous extract of Cinnamomum zeylanicum on non-transgenic Alzheimer's disease rat model: Biochemical, histological, and behavioural studies, *Nutr Neurosci*, 16, 1-12

Page 81   81 Solfrizzi V et al, 2015, Coffee Consumption Habits and the Risk of Mild Cognitive Impairment: The Italian Longitudinal Study on Aging. *J Alzheimers Dis*, 47, 4, 889-99

82 Lee M et al, 2016, Quercetin, not caffeine, is a major neuroprotective component in coffee, *Neurobiol Aging*, 46, 113-123

83 Nakagawa T et al, 2016, Improvement of memory recall by quercetin in rodent contextual fear conditioning and human early-stage Alzheimer's disease patients, *Neuroreport*, 27, 9, 671-6

84 Lin J et al, 2005, Green tea polyphenols epigallocatechin gallate inhibits adipogenesis and induces apoptosis in 3T3-L1 adipocytes, *Obes Res*, 13, 6, 982-90

Page 82   85 Lin J et al, 2005, Green tea polyphenols epigallocatechin gallate inhibits adipogenesis and induces apoptosis in 3T3-L1 adipocytes, *Obes Res*, 13, 6, 982-90

86 Ronan L et al, 2016, Obesity associated with increased brain-age from mid-life, *Neurobiology of Aging*, DOI: http://dx.doi.org/10.1016/j.neurobiolaging.2016.07.010

87 Mandel SA et al, 2011, Understanding the broad-spectrum neuroprotective action profile ofgreen tea polyphenols in aging and neurodegenerative diseases, *J Alzheimers Dis*, 25, 2, 187-208

Page 83   88 Gella A, Durany N, 2009, Oxidative stress in Alzheimer disease, *Cell Adh Migr, 3*, 1, 88-93

89 Yuan T et al, 2016, Pomegranate's Neuroprotective Effects against Alzheimer's Disease Ar Mediated by Urolithins, Its Ellagitannin-Gut Microbial Derived Metabolites. *ACS Chem Neurosci*, 7, 1, 26-33

90 Calder PC et al, 2009, Inflammatory disease processes and interactions with nutrition, *B J Nutr*, 101, Supp 1-45

Chapter 6

Page 84   91 Fontana L et al, 2006, Long-term low-protein, low-calorie diet and endurance exercise modulate metabolic factors associated with cancer risk, *Am J Clin Nutr*, 84, 6, 1456-62

Page 85   92 Horne BD et al, 2015, Health effects of intermittent fasting: hormesis or harm? A systematic review, *Am J Clin Nutr*, 102, 2, 464-70.

Page 86   93 Jaeger PA, Wyss-Coray T, 2009, All-you-can-eat: autophagy in neurodegeneration and neuroprotection. *Mol Neurodegener.* 4:16.

Page 87   94 Daulatzai MA, 2015, Non-celiac gluten sensitivity triggers gut dysbiosis, neuroinflammation, gut-brain axis dysfunction, and vulnerability for dementia. *CNS Neurol Disord Drug Targets*, 14, 1, 110-31

           95 Meijer CR et al, 2015, Coeliac disease and noncoeliac gluten sensitivity, *J Pediatr Gastroenterol Nutr.* 2015 Apr;60(4):429-32.

           96 Hogg-Kollars S et al, 2011, Gluten sensitivity a new condition in the spectrum of gluten-related disorders, *Complete Nutrition*, 11, 4, July/August

Chapter 7

Page 89   97 Romaquera D, 2013, Consumption of sweet beverages and type 2 diabetes incidence in European adults: results from EPIC-InterAct, *Diabetologia*, 56, 7, 1520-30

           98 Fagherazzi G et al, 2013, Consumption of artificially and sugar-sweetened beverages and incident type 2 diabetes in the Etude Epidémiologique auprès des femmes de la Mutuelle Générale de l'Education Nationale–European Prospective Investigation into Cancer and Nutrition cohort, *Am J Clin Nutr*, 97, 3, 571-23

           99 McNay E, presented at the Annual Society for Neuroscience meeting in San Diego, USA, December 2013

Page 90   100 De la Monte S and Wands JR, 2005, Review of insulin and insulin-like growth factor expression, signaling and malfunction in the central nervous system: Relevance to Alzheimer's disease, *Journal of Alzheimer's Disease*, 7, 1, 45-61

Page 90   101 Crane PK et al, 2013, Glucose levels and risk of dementia, *Eng J Med*, 369, 6, 540-8

Page 96   102 Teff KL et al, 2009, Endocrine and metabolic effects of consuming fructose- and glucosesweetened beverages with meals in obese men and women: influence of insulin resistance on plasma triglyceride responses, *J Clin Endocrinol Metab*, 94, 5, 1562-9

Page 98   103 Feijo Fde M et al, 2013, Saccharin and aspartame, compared with sucrose, induce greater weight gain in adult Wistar rats, at similar total caloric intake levels, *Appetite*, 60, 1, 203-7

          104 Hazuda H et al, presented at the American Diabetes Association's Scientific Sessions, San Diego, 2011

Chapter 8

Page 99   105 *The Independent Food Commission's Food Magazine* 2005

Page 100 106 Schaefer EJ et al, 2006, Plasma phosphatidylcholine docosahexaenoic acid content and risk of dementia and Alzheimer disease: the Framingham Heart Study. *Arch Neurol*, 63, 11, 1545-1550

          107 Arab L et al, 2010, Are certain lifestyle habits associated with lower Alzheimer's disease risk? *J Alzheimer's Dis*, 20, 3, 785-794

          108 Ma QL et al, 2007, Omega 3 fatty acid docosahexaenoic acid increases SorLA/LR11, a sorting protein with reduced expression in sporadic Alzheimer's disease (AD): relevance to AD prevention, *J Neurosci*, 27, 52, 14299-307

Page 101 109 Pottala J et al, 2014, Higher RBC EPA + DHA corresponds with larger total brain and hippocampal volumes: WHIMS-MRI study. *Neurology*, 82(5):435-42

          110 Lavie C, 2009, Omega 3 polyunsaturated fatty acids and cardiovascular diseases, *Journal of the American College of Cardiology*, 54, 7, 585-94

          111 The Preventable Causes of Death in the United States: Comparative Risk Assessment of Dietary, Lifestyle, and Metabolic Risk Factors" stud, April 2009, *PLoS Medicine*

Chapter 8

Page 101 112 Simopoulos AO, 1991, Omega 3 fatty acids in health and
disease and in growth and development, *Am J Clin Nutr*, 54:
438-463 and Meyer BJ et al, 2003, Dietary intakes and food
sources of omega 6 and omega 3 polyunsaturated fatty acids,
Lipids, 38, 4, 391-8

Page 102 113 Simopoulos AP, 2016, An Increase in the Omega 6/Omega 3
Fatty Acid Ratio Increases the Risk for Obesity, *Nutrients*, 8, 3,
128

114 Daley C et al, 2010, A review of fatty acid profiles and
antioxidant content in grass fed and grainfed beef, *Nutrition
Journal*, 9, 10 and Ponnampalam EN et al, 2006, Effect of
feeding systems on omega 3 fatty acids, conjugated linoleic
acid and trans fatty acids in Australian beef cuts: potential
impact on human health, *Asia Pac J Clin Nutr*, 15, 1, 21-9

Page 105 115 Ramprasath VR et al, 2013, Enhanced increase of omega 3
index in healthy individuals with response to 4-week n-3
fatty acid supplementation from krill oil versus fish oil.
Lipids Health Dis, 12, 178

Page 106 116 Nichols PD et al, 2014, Commentary on a trial comparing
krill oil versus fish oil. *Lipids Health Dis*,13, 2

117 Salem N, Kuratko CN, 2014, A reexamination of krill oil
bioavailability studies. *Lipids Health Dis*, 13, 137

118 Yurko-Mauro K et al, 2015, Similar eicosapentaenoic acid
and docosahexaenoic acid plasma levels achieved with
fish oil or krill oil in a randomized double-blind four-week
bioavailability study. *Lipids in Health and Disease*, 14, 99

Page 107 119 Seshadri S et al, 2002, Plasma homocysteine as a risk factor
for dementia and Alzheimer's disease, *NEJM*, 346, 7,476-483

120 Douaud G et al, 2013, Preventing Alzheimer's disease-related
gray matter atrophy by B vitamin treatment, *PNAS*, 110, 23,
9523-9528

121 Smith AD et al, 2010, Homocysteine-lowering by B vitamins
slows the rate of accelerated brain atrophy in mild cognitive
impairment: a randomised controlled trial, *PloS One*, 5, 9,
e12244

Page 108 122 Jerneren F et al, 2015, Brain atrophy in cognitively impaired elderly: the importance of long-chain ω-3 fatty acids and B vitamin status in a randomized controlled trial, *Am J Clin Nutr*, 102, 1, 215-21

123 Oulhaj A et al, 2016, Omega 3 Fatty Acid Status Enhances the Prevention of Cognitive Decline by B Vitamins in Mild Cognitive Impairment. *J Alzheimers Dis*, 50, 2, 547-57

Page 110 124 http://www.nchpeg.org/nutrition/index.php?option=com_content&view=article&id=454&tmpl=compone nt

125 Rai V, 2016, Methylenetetrahydrofolate Reductase (MTHFR) C677T Polymorphism andAlzheimer Disease Risk: a Meta-Analysis, *Mol Neurobiol*, Jan 28. [Epub ahead of print]

126 Hu J et al, 2016, Intake and Biomarkers of Folate and Risk of Cancer Morbidity in Older Adults, NHANES 1999-2002 with Medicare Linkage. *PLoS One*, Feb 10, 11, 2

Page 111 127 Paul V and Ekambaram P, 2011, Involvement of nitric oxide in learning and memory processes, *Indian J Med Res*, 133, 5, 471-478)

128 Jing Y et al, 2009, L-arginine and Alzheimer's Disease, *Int J Clin Exp Pathol*, 2,3, 211-238

129 Ohtsuka Y and Nakaya J, 2000, Effect of oral administration of L-arginine on senile dementia, *Am J Med*, 108, 5, 439

130 Bianchetti A et al, 2003, Effects of Acetyl-L-Carnitine In Alzheimer's Disease Patients Unresponsive to Acetylcholinesterase Inhibitors, *Curr Med Res Opin*, 19, 4, 350-3

131 Cristofano A et al, 2016, Serum Levels of Acyl-Carnitines along the Continuum from Normal toAlzheimer's Dementia, *PLoS One*, 11, 5, e)155694

Page 112 132 Bianchetti A et al, 2003, Effects of Acetyl-L-Carnitine In Alzheimer's Disease Patients Unresponsive to Acetylcholinesterase Inhibitors, *Curr Med Res Opin*, 19, 4, 350-3

133 Holmquist L et al, 2007, Lipoic acid as a novel treatment for Alzheimer's disease and related dementias. *Pharmacol Ther.* 113, 1,154-64

Chapter 8

Page 112 134 El Midaoui A and de Champlain J, 2002, Prevention of hypertension, insulin resistance and oxidative stress by alpha-lipoic acid, *Hypertension*, 39, 2, 303-7

135 Chung SY et al, 1995, Administration of phosphatidylcholine increases brain acetylcholine concentration and improves memory in mice with dementia, *J Nutr*, 125, 6, 1484-9

136 Ko M et al, 2016, Phosphatidylcholine protects neurons from toxic effects of amyloid β-protein in culture, *Brain Res*, 1642, 376-83

137 Qu MH et al, 2016, Docosahexaenoic Acid-Phosphatidylcholine Improves Cognitive Deficits in an Aβ3-35-Induced Alzheimer's Disease Rat Model, *Cur Top Med Chem*, 16, 5, 558-64

Page 113 138 Zhang YY et al, 2015, Effect of phosphatidylserine on memory in patients and rats withAlzheimer's disease, *Genet Mol Res*, 14, 3, 9325-33

139 Vakhapova V et al, 2010, Phosphatidylserine containing omega 3 fatty acids may improve memory abilities in non-demented elderly with memory complaints: a double-blind placebo-controlled trial, *Dement Geriatr Cogn Disord*, 29, 5, 467-74

140 Suchy J et al, 2009, Dietary supplementation with a combination of alpha-lipoic acid, acetyl-Lcarnitine, glycerophosphocoline, docosahexaenoic acid, and phosphatidylserine reduces oxidative damage to murine brain and improves cognitive performance, *Nutr Res*, 29, 1, 70-4

141 Brewer GJ, Kaur S, 2013, Zinc deficiency and zinc therapy efficacy with reduction of serum free copper in Alzheimer's disease, *Int J Alzheimers Dis*, 586365

Page 114 142 Brewer GJ, 2014, Alzheimer's disease causation by copper toxicity and treatment with zinc. *Front Aging Neurosci*, 6, 92

Page 115 143 Littlejohns T et al, 2014, Vitamin D and the risk of dementia and Alzheimer disease. *Neurology*, 83, 10, 920-928

Page 116 144 Darup D et al, 2012, A reverse J-shaped association of all-cause mortality with serum 25-hydroxyvitamin D in general practice: the CopD study, J Clin Endocrinol, *Metab*, 97, 8, 2644-52

145 Hyponnen E et al, 2009, Serum 25-hydroxyvitamin D and IgE - a significant but nonlinear relationship. *Allergy*, 54, 4, 613-620

146 Banerjee A et al, 2015, Vitamin D and Alzheimer's Disease: Neurocognition to Therapeutics, *Int J Alzheimer's Dis*, 2015, ID 192747

147 Heaney RP et al, 2011, Vitamin D(3) is more potent than vitamin D(2) in humans. *J Clin Endocrinol Metab*, 96, 3, E447-52

Page 117 148 Zandi PP et al, 2004, Reduced risk of Alzheimer disease in users of antioxidant vitamin supplements: the Cache County Study.*Arch Neurol*. 2004 Jan;61(1):82-8.

149 Kook SY et al, 2014, High-dose of vitamin C supplementation reduces amyloid plaque burden and ameliorates pathological changes in the brain of 5XFAD mice. *Cell Death Dis*. 2014 Feb 27;5:e1083

Page 118 150 Afkhami-Ardekani M, Shoiaoddiny-Ardekani A, 2007, Effect of vitamin C on blood glucose, serum lipids & serum insulin in type 2 diabetes patients. *Indian J Med Res*, 26, 5, 471-4

151 Turner RS et al, 2015, A randomized, double-blind, placebo-controlled trial of resveratrol forAlzheimer disease. *Neurology*, 85, 16, 1383-91,

Page 119 152 Fadl NN et al, 2013, Serrapeptase and nattokinase intervention for relieving Alzheimer'sdisease pathophysiology in rat model. *Hum Exp Toxicol*, 32, 7, 721-35

153 Kern J et al, 2016, Calcium supplementation and risk of dementia in women with cerebrovascular disease. *Neurology*, August, (Epub ahead of print)

Page 120 154 Bolland M et al, 2010, Effect of calcium supplements on risk of myocardial infarction and cardiovascular events: meta-analysis, *BMJ*, 341, c3691

155 Galland L, 2014, The gut microbiome and the brain. *J Med Food*, 12, 1261-72

Chapter 8

Page 121 156 Isolauri E, Salminen S, Probiotics: use in allergic disorders: a Nutrition, Allergy, Mucosal Immunology, and Intestinal Microbiota (NAMI) Research Group Report. *J Clin Gastroenterol.* 2008 Jul: 42 Suppl 2:S91-6)

157 Calder PC et al, Inflammatory disease processes and interactions with nutrition, 2009, *B J Nutr*, 101, Supp 1-45

158 Tang ML et al, Probiotics and prebiotics: clinical effects in allergic disease. *Curr Opin Pediatr*, 22, 5, 626-34

159 DiBaise JK et al, Gut microbiota and its possible relationship with obesity. *Mayo Clin Proc*, 2008 Ar;83(4):460-9

160 Cani PD et al, 2008, Role of gut microflora in the development of obesity and insulin resistance following high-fat diet feeding. *Pathol Biol (Paris)*, 56(5):305-9

161 Ridaura VK et al, 2013, Gut microbiota from twins discordant for obesity modulate metabolism in mice. *Science*, 341, 6150, 1241214

Page 122 162 Nickerson KP et al, 2014, The dietary polysaccharide maltodextrin promotes Salmonella survival and mucosal colonization in mice, *PLoS One*, 9, 7

Page 123 163 Mori K et al, 2011, Effects of Hericium erinaceus on amyloid β(25-35) peptide-induced learning and memory deficits in mice, Biomed Res, 32, 1, 67-72

164 Mori K et al, 2009, Improving effects of the mushroom Yamabushitake (Hericium erinaceus) on mild cognitive impairment: a double-blind placebo-controlled clinical trial, *Phytother Res*, 23, 3, 367-72

165 Trovato A et al, 2016, Redox modulation of cellular stress response and lipoxin A4 expression by Hericium Erinaceus in rat brain: relevance to Alzheimer's disease pathogenesis. *Immun Ageing*, 13, 23

166 Tzeng T-T et al, 2016, Erinacine A-enriched Hericium erinaceusmycelium ameliorates Alzheimer's disease-related pathologies in APPswe/PS1dE9 transgenic mice, *J Biomed Sci*, 23, 49

Page 123 167 Yang G et al, 2016, Ginkgo Biloba for Mild Cognitive Impairment and Alzheimer's Disease: A Systematic Review and Meta-Analysis of Randomized Controlled Trials. *Curr Top Med Chem*, 16, 5, 520-8

Page 124 168 Goozee KG et al, 2016, Examining the potential clinical value of curcumin in the prevention and diagnosis of Alzheimer's disease, *Br J Nutr*, 115, 3, 449-65

169 Findings presented at the British Psychological Society Conference in Nottingham, April 2016

170 Ozaroawski M et al, 2013, Rosmarinus officinalis L. leaf extract improves memory impairment and affects acetylcholinesterase and butyrylcholinesterase activities in rat brain. *Fitoterapia*, 91, 261-71

171 Rasoolijazi H et al, 2015, The effect of rosemary extract on spatial memory, learning and antioxidant enzymes activities in the hippocampus of middle-aged rats. *Med J Islam Repub Iran*, 29, 187

Page 125 172 Findings presented at the British Psychological Society Conference in Nottingham, April 2016

Chapter 9

Page 128 173 Ronan L et al, 2016, Obesity associated with increased brain-age from mid-life, *Neurobiology of Aging*, DOI: http://dx.doi.org/10.1016/j.neurobiolaging.2016.07.010

Page 129 174 Whitmer RA et al, 2008, Central obesity and increased risk od dementia more than three decades later, *Neurology*, 71, 14, 1057-64

Page 130 175 Nouchi R et al, 2014, Four weeks of combination exercise training improved executive functions, episodic memory, and processing speed in healthy elderly people: evidence from a randomized controlled trial. *Age* 36, 2, 787-99

176 Colcombe S, Kramer AF. Fitness effects on the cognitive function of older adults: a meta-analytic study. *Psychol Sci.* 2003;14(2):125-130.

177 Eyre HA et al, 2016, Changes in Neural Connectivity and Memory Following a Yoga Intervention for Older Adults: A Pilot Study, *J Alzheimer's Dis*, 52, 2, 673-84

Chapter 9

Page 131   178 Erickson KI et al, 2014, Physical activity, fitness, and gray matter volume. Neurobiol Aging, 35, *Suppl 2*, S20-8

179 Wright H and Jenks RA, 2016, Sex on the brain! Associations between sexual activity and cognitive function in older age., *Age Ageing*, 45, 2, 313-7

Chapter 10

Page 132   180 Johansson L et al, 2013, Common psychosocial stressors in middleaged women related to longstanding distress and increased risk of Alzheimer's disease: a 38-year longitudinal population study, *BMJ Open*, 3, 9, e003142

Page 135   181 Britta K et al, 2011, Mindfulness practice leads to increases in regional brain gray matter density, *Psychiatry Res*, 191, 1, 36-43

Page 136   182 Kang JE et al, 2009, Amyloid-beta dynamics are regulated by orexin and the sleep-wake cycle. *Science*. 326, 5955, 1005-1007.

183 Spira AP, et al, 2013, Self-reported Sleep and β-Amyloid Deposition in Community-Dwelling Older Adults, *JAMA Neurol*, 70, 12, 1537-43.

Page 137   184 Lee H et al, 2015, The effect of body posture on brain glymphatic transport, *J Neurosci*, 35, 31, 111034-44

185 Gooley JJ et al, 2010, Spectral responses of the human circadian system depend on the irradiance and duration of exposure to light. *Sci Transl Med*, 2, 31, 31ra33

186 Gooley JJ et al, 2011, Exposure to room light before bedtime suppresses melatonin onset and shortens melatonin duration in humans. *J Clin Endocrinol Metab*, 96, 3, E463-72

187 Mukda S et al, 2016, Melatonin administration reverses the alteration of amyloid precursor protein-cleaving secretases expression in aged mouse hippocampus, *Neurosci Lett*, 621, 39-46

Page 138   188 Karami Z et al, 2016, Effect of Daylight on Melatonin and Subjective General Health Factors in Elderly People. *Iran J Public Health*, 45, 5, 636-43

Page 140 189 Deng M, Wang XF, 2016, Acupuncture for amnestic mild cognitive impairment: a meta-analysis of randomised controlled trials, *Acupunct Med*, August 4 (Epub ahead of print), doi: 10.1136/acupmed-2015-010989

Chapter 11

Page 142 190 Yumoto, S et al, 2009, Demonstration of aluminum in amyloid fibers in the cores of senile plaques in the brains of patients with Alzheimer's disease. *Journal of Inorganic Biochemistry*. 103 (11): 1579–84.

191 Kawahara M, 2016, Link between aluminium neurotoxicity and neurodegenerative disorders, *Nihon Rinsho*, 74, 7, 1176-85

Page 143 192 Kawahara M, 2005, Effects of aluminium on the nervous system and its possible link with neurodegenerative diseases. *J Alzheimers Dis*, 8, 2, 171-82

193 Tomlienovic L, 2011, Aluminium and Alzheimer's disease: after a century of controversy, is there a plausible link? *J Alzheimers Dis*, 23, 4, 567-98.

194 Mutter J et al, 2010, Does inorganic mercury play a role in Alzheimer's disease? *J Alzheimers Dis*. 22(2):357-374.

Page 144 195 Morris MC et al, 2016, Association of Seafood Consumption, Brain Mercury Level, and APOE ε4 Status With Brain Neuropathology in Older Adults, *JAMA*, 315, 5, 489-97

196 Kroger E, Laforce R, 2016, Fish Consumption, Brain Mercury, and Neuropathology in Patients With Alzheimer Disease and Dementia, *JAMA*, 315, 5, 465-466

Page 145 197 Richardson JR et al, 2014, Elevated serum pesticide levels and risk for Alzheimer disease, *JAMA Neurol*, 71, 3, 284-90

198 Baldi I et al, 2003, Neurodegenerative diseases and exposure to pesticides in the elderly., *Epidemiol*, 157, 5, 409-414

199 Parron T et al, 2011, Association between environmental exposure to pesticides and neurodegenerative diseases, *Toxicol Appl Pharmacol*, 256, 3, 379-83

200 Palmer MJ et al, 2013, Cholinergic pesticides cause mushroom body neuronal inactivation in honeybees, *Nat Commun*, 4, 1634

Chapter 11

Page 146 201 Hautot D et al, 2003, Preliminary evaluation of nanoscale biogenic magnetite in Alzheimer's disease brain tissue, Proc R Soc Lond B (Suppl) 270, S62-S64 With Alzheimer Disease and Dementia, *JAMA*, 315, 5, 465-466

202 Maher B et al, 2016, Magnetite pollution nanoparticles in the human brain, *PNAS*, 113, 39, 10797-10801

203 Weiss B, 2007, Can Endocrine Disruptors Influence Neuroplasticity In The Aging Brain? *Neurotoxicology*, 28, 5, 938-950

Page 147 204 Haiszan T, Leranth C, 2010, Bisphenol A interferes with synaptic remodelling, *Front Neuroendocrinol*, 31, 4, 519-30

205 https://www.niehs.nih.gov/health/topics/agents/sya-bpa/

Page 149 206 S Sabia et al, 2014, Alcohol consumption and cognitive decline in early old age, *Neurology*, 82, 332-339

207 Stavro K et al, 2013, Widespread and sustained cognitive deficits in alcoholism: a meta-analysis, *Addict Biol*, 18, 2, 201-13

Chapter 12

Page 151 208 Riley KP et al, 2005, Early life linguistic ability, late life cognitive function, and neuropathology: findings from the Nun Study, *Neurobiology of Aging*, 26, 3, 341-347

Page 152 209 Verghese J et al, 2003, Leisure activities and the risk of dementia in the elderly. *N Eng J Med*, 348, 25, 2508-16

210 Hall CB et al, 2009, Cognitive activities delay onset of memory decline in persons who develop dementia, *Neurology*, 73, 5, 356-61

211 Pillai JA et al, 2011, Association of crossword puzzle participation with memory decline in persons who develop dementia, *J Int Neuropsychol Soc*, 17, 6, 1006-13

Page 153 212 Rebok GW et al, 2014, Ten-year effects of the advanced cognitive training for independent and vital elderly cognitive training trial on cognition and everyday functioning in older adults, *J Am Geriatr Soc*, 62, 1, 16-24. Edwards JD et al, 2016, The ACTIVE Study: What We Have Learned and What Is Next? Cognitive Training Reduces Incident Dementia Across Ten Years, presented at the Alzheimer's Association International Conference in Toronto, August 2016

Page 153 213 A Consensus on the Brain Training Industry from the Scientific Community, Max Planck Institute for Human Development and Stanford Centre on Longevity, October 2014

Page 155 214 Alladi S et al, 2013, Bilingualism delays age of onset of dementia, independent of education and immigration status, *Neurology*, 81, 22, 1938-44

215 Bak TH et al, 2014, Does bilingualism influence cognitive ageing, *Ann Neurol*, 75, 6, 959-63

216 Abutalebi J et al, 2015, Bilingualism provides a neural reserve for aging populations. *Neuropsycholoiga*, 69, 201-10

217 Balbag MA et al, 2014, Playing a Musical Instrument as a Protective Factor against Dementia and Cognitive Impairment: A Population-Based Twin Study, *Int J Alzheimer's Dis*, 2014:836748

218 Palisson J et al, 2015, Music enhances verbal episodic memory in Alzheimer's disease, *J Clin Exp Neuropsychol*, 37, 5, 503-17

Chapter 13

Page 158 219 Fiandaca MS et al, 2015, Identification of preclinical Alzheimer's disease by a profile of pathogenic proteins in neurally derived blood exosomes: A case-control study, *Azheimer's Dement*, 11, 6, 600-7

220 Kapogiannis D et al, 2015, Dysfunctionally phosphorylated type 1 insulin receptor substrate in neural-derived blood exosomes of preclinical Alzheimer's disease, *FASEB J*, 29, 2, 589-96

221 Fiandaca MS et al, 2015, Plasma 24-metabolite Panel Predicts Preclinical Transition to Clinical Stages of Alzheimer's Disease, *Front Neurol*, 6, 237

Page 161 222 Seshadri S et al, 2002, Plasma homocysteine as a risk factor for dementia and Alzheimer's disease, *NEJM*, 346, 7,476-483

Page 162 223 Brudnak MA, 2002, Probiotics as an adjuvant to detoxification protocols, *Med Hypotheses*, 58, 5, 382-5

Page 165 224 Pirastu N et al, 2014, European Human Genetics Conference

Chapter 13

Page 168 225 Ngandu T et al, 2015, A 2 year multidomain intervention of diet, exercise, cognitive training, and vascular risk monitoring versus control to prevent cognitive decline in at-risk elderly people (FINGER): a randomised controlled trial. *Lancet*, 385, 9984, 2255-63

226 Bredesen DE et al, 2016, Reversal of cognitive decline in Alzheimer's disease. *Aging (Albany NY)*, 8, 6, 1250-8

Page 169 227 Merrill DA et al, 2016, Modifiable Risk Factors and Brain Positron Emission Tomography Measures of Amyloid and Tau in Nondemented Adults with Mcmory Complaints, *The American Journal of Geriatric Psychiatry*, 24, 9, 729-737

INDEX